The content of this book is based on various sources and is intended for
educational and entertainment purposes only. While the author has
made every effort to ensure the accuracy, completeness, and reliability of
the information provided, the information may be subject to errors,
omissions, or inaccuracies. Therefore, the author makes no warranties,
express or implied, regarding the content of this book.

Readers are advised to seek the guidance of a licensed professional before
attempting any techniques or actions outlined in this book. The author is
not responsible for any losses, damages, or injuries that may arise from
the use of information contained within. The information provided in
this book is not intended to be a substitute for professional advice, and
readers should not rely solely on the information presented.

By reading this book, readers acknowledge that the author is not
providing legal, financial, medical, or professional advice. Any reliance
on the information contained in this book is solely at the reader's own
risk.

*Thank you for selecting this book as a valuable source of knowledge and
inspiration. Our aim is to provide you with insights and information
that will enrich your understanding and enhance your personal growth.
We appreciate your decision to embark on this journey of discovery
with us, and we hope that this book will exceed your expectations and
leave a lasting impact on your life.*

Title: Born to Run-Inside the World of Greyhound Racing
Subtitle: The Thrills, Passions and Ethics Behind a Storied Sport

Author: William R. Foster

Table of Contents

Introduction **6**

A Brief History of Greyhound Racing 6

Greyhounds Through the Ages - Their Abilities and Role in Society 9

The Rise of Modern Commercial Dog Racing 12

Overview of the Book's Scope and Purpose 15

Chapter 1: The Origins of Greyhound Racing **18**

Ancient Roots and Early Appearances in History 18

Import to America and Early US Racing 20

Emergence of Organized Tracks and Professional Kennels ... 23

Spread of Popularity Across Post-War America 25

Greyhound Racing's Golden Age 28

Chapter 2: The Basics of the Sport **31**

Types of Races and Track Configurations 31

Attributes of Successful Racing Greyhounds 34

Training Regimens and Exercise Routines 37

Racing Strategies and Techniques 40

Rules and Regulations of Races 44

Chapter 3: A Day at the Racetrack **47**

Arriving at the Track and Reading the Program 47

Wagering - How to Bet on the Dogs 50

Pregame Rituals and Trackside Traditions 56

The Race Experience - Following the Mechanical Lure 61

Behind the Scenes - Life in the Racing Kennels 66

Chapter 4: Major Races and Champions **71**

The Sport's Classic Races and Prizes 71

Notable Racetracks that Host Premier Events 76

Hall of Fame Greyhounds Through History 82

Profiles of Top Racers from Past Eras 86

Current Rising Stars and Fan Favorites................................ *90*

Chapter 5: Controversies and Animal Welfare 94

Injuries and Health Issues for Racing Greyhounds *94*

Scientific Studies on Breed Welfare.................................... *98*

Doping Scandals and Prevention Efforts..........................*102*

Ethics of Breeding Practices and Culling *107*

Retirement and Adoption of Former Racers *112*

Chapter 6: Greyhound Breeding and Bloodlines 117

Desirable Qualities in Racing Greyhounds...........................*117*

Selective Breeding Practices Over Time...............................*122*

Top Breeders and Kennel Lineages...................................*127*

Contribution of Genetics vs. Training *132*

Future of Selective Breeding in the Sport............................*136*

Chapter 7: Owners, Trainers, and Handlers............140

Leading Owners and Racing Syndicates *140*

Famous Trainers and Their Methods.................................*145*

Handlers and Their Relationships with Dogs.......................*149*

Rags to Riches Stories of Success *154*

Rising Personalities to Watch *158*

Chapter 8: The Business of Dog Racing...................162

Economics of the Racing Industry *162*

Media Deals and Broadcasting *167*

Gambling and Bookmaking..*171*

Regulation and State Oversight *175*

Challenges from Animal Rights Groups *179*

Chapter 9: Greyhound Racing by Region..................183

The Sport's Roots in Florida and the South *183*

Tracks and Styles Across the Western US.............................*186*

Midwestern Racing Heritage and Culture *189*

New England's Connections to Greyhound Racing..................*192*

International Racing in the UK, Ireland, Australia *195*

Chapter 10: The Future of Greyhound Racing 198

Changing Public Perceptions and Ethical Concerns.............198

Shifting Legislative Landscape and Regulations 202

Potential Safety and Welfare Reforms.................................. 206

Adapting the Sport to New Technologies.............................210

Preserving Racing's Traditions in Tomorrow's World 215

Conclusion... 220

Key Takeaways and Insights from the World of Greyhound
Racing 220

Reflections on the Sport's History and Future..................... 226

Parting Thoughts on the Lives of Racing Greyhounds......... 230

Final Remarks on the Book's Chronicling of This World 234

Wordbook..238

Supplementary Materials 241

Introduction
A Brief History of Greyhound Racing

Greyhound racing, a sport of speed, skill, and grace, has a rich history woven into the fabric of human civilization. As we embark on this journey through the world of greyhound racing in "Born to Run," it is essential to delve into the roots of this captivating sport.

The origins of greyhound racing trace back to ancient civilizations, where the swift and agile hounds were revered for their hunting prowess. In the annals of history, depictions of greyhounds have been discovered in Egyptian tombs, emphasizing their esteemed role in society. These early records provide a glimpse into a time when these dogs were cherished companions and valued for their exceptional abilities.

The transition of greyhounds from revered companions to racing competitors is a testament to their innate qualities. In the United States, the sport found its footing in the early 20th century, as informal races between dog owners evolved into organized events. The emergence of dedicated tracks and kennels marked a pivotal moment, transforming greyhound racing into a professional and regulated sport.

Post-war America witnessed the rapid spread of greyhound racing's popularity, capturing the imagination of a nation eager for entertainment and excitement. The golden age of the sport saw the establishment of iconic tracks and the rise of legendary greyhounds that etched their names into the annals of racing history.

The Basics of the Sport (Chapter 2) delve deeper into the types of races, attributes of successful racing greyhounds, and the intricate training regimens that propel these dogs to extraordinary speeds. It explores the nuances of racing, from strategies on the track to the rules and regulations that govern each race.

As we journey through this exploration of greyhound racing, it is crucial to understand the sport's foundations and how it has evolved over centuries. The allure of the mechanical lure and the pulse-pounding excitement of the race experience are integral to the narrative, providing readers with a visceral understanding of what makes greyhound racing a captivating spectacle.

In subsequent chapters, we will unravel the stories of major races and champions (Chapter 4), confront controversies and delve into the realm of animal welfare (Chapter 5), and explore the intricate world of breeding and bloodlines (Chapter 6). We will meet the key players — owners, trainers, and handlers (Chapter 7) — who shape the destiny of these magnificent athletes.

The journey through greyhound racing extends beyond the tracks, delving into the business aspects (Chapter 8) and examining the regional influences that have shaped the sport's identity (Chapter 9). As we peer into the future (Chapter 10), we will explore the shifting landscape of public perceptions, legislative changes, and the ongoing efforts to ensure the safety and welfare of these remarkable athletes.

In this exploration of "Born to Run," we invite you to immerse yourself in the world of greyhound racing — a world where speed meets strategy, and the bond between human and hound creates a tapestry of stories that transcend time. The greyhound, born to run, takes center stage, and through these pages, their legacy unfolds.

Greyhounds Through the Ages - Their Abilities and Role in Society

As we explore the pages of "Born to Run - Inside the World of Greyhound Racing," it is paramount to delve into the historical tapestry that weaves together the abilities and societal roles of the greyhound. These sleek and elegant canines have left an indelible mark on civilizations throughout the ages, their prowess extending far beyond the racetrack.

In the annals of ancient history, greyhounds emerge as revered companions, valued for their unique blend of speed, agility, and intelligence. The roots of this bond between humans and greyhounds can be traced back to civilizations such as ancient Egypt, where depictions in hieroglyphics and tomb paintings showcase these canines in roles that transcend mere utility. In this era, greyhounds were not merely hunting companions; they were symbols of grace, loyalty, and nobility.

The Greeks, recognizing the extraordinary athleticism of greyhounds, incorporated them into their mythology. These canines became associated with the gods, symbols of swiftness and grace. This cultural integration elevated the status of greyhounds, positioning them as creatures of beauty and divine significance.

As societies evolved, so did the roles of greyhounds. In medieval Europe, these dogs were the favored hunting companions of the aristocracy. Their speed and keen eyesight made them indispensable in pursuing game, a role that further solidified their place among the elite. Paintings from this period depict greyhounds in regal settings, a testament to their esteemed status.

The Renaissance saw a shift in the perception of greyhounds. No longer confined to the elite, these canines found a place in the homes of the burgeoning middle class. Their companionship was cherished, and their innate hunting abilities were adapted for new roles, including coursing competitions that pitted them against each other in friendly contests of speed and skill.

The transition from hunting to racing marked a pivotal moment in the history of greyhounds. In the early 20th century, particularly in the United States, informal races between dog owners laid the groundwork for the emergence of organized racing. The inherent speed and grace of greyhounds became the focal point, captivating the public and setting the stage for the development of professional tracks and kennels.

Chapter 1 explores these ancient roots and early appearances in history, providing a foundation for understanding how greyhounds evolved from revered companions to racing competitors. From ancient Egypt to medieval Europe, the journey of the greyhound is a testament to their adaptability and enduring appeal.

In the chapters to come, we will witness the rise of modern commercial dog racing, explore the intricacies of the sport in "The Basics of the Sport" (Chapter 2), and experience a day at the racetrack in Chapter 3. The narrative will unfold, tracing the lineage of major races and champions (Chapter 4), addressing controversies and the critical issue of animal welfare (Chapter 5), and unraveling the complex world of greyhound breeding and bloodlines (Chapter 6).

The greyhound, a companion to pharaohs, a symbol of nobility, and now a racing champion, has transitioned through the ages, leaving an indelible mark on the hearts of those who have witnessed their remarkable journey. In the chapters that follow, we will continue to explore the multifaceted world of greyhound racing, where history, athleticism, and the enduring bond between human and hound converge.

The Rise of Modern Commercial Dog Racing

In the expansive landscape of "Born to Run - Inside the World of Greyhound Racing," a pivotal chapter unfolds in the narrative: the rise of modern commercial dog racing. This transformative era saw the evolution of greyhound racing from informal contests into a highly organized and commercially driven sport that captivated the masses.

As we navigate through this historical juncture, it becomes evident that the roots of modern greyhound racing extend deep into the early 20th century. The United States played a central role in this evolution, with informal races among dog owners laying the foundation for a burgeoning industry. These early races, often impromptu and held in open fields, foreshadowed the organized events that would soon define the sport.

The emergence of organized tracks marked a significant shift in the trajectory of greyhound racing. These purpose-built venues provided a structured environment for races, enhancing the spectator experience and contributing to the professionalization of the sport. The establishment of these tracks was not merely a logistical development but a cultural one, symbolizing the formalization of greyhound racing as a legitimate form of entertainment.

Parallel to the growth of tracks, professional kennels began to take shape. Skilled trainers and handlers entered the scene, recognizing the potential of greyhounds as competitive athletes. The systematic training regimens employed by these professionals contributed to the refinement of racing techniques, propelling the sport into a new era of competitiveness.

The spread of popularity across post-war America was a testament to the sport's appeal. Greyhound racing became a staple in communities, drawing crowds eager for excitement and spectacle. The golden age of greyhound racing was characterized by a proliferation of tracks and a surge in the number of racing greyhounds, each vying for glory on the tracks that had become iconic symbols of this burgeoning industry.

Chapter 1, which explores the origins of greyhound racing, lays the groundwork for understanding this transformative period. From ancient roots to early appearances in history and the importation of the sport to America, the journey to modern commercial dog racing is a testament to the adaptability of greyhounds and the human fascination with their extraordinary abilities.

As we delve into the subsequent chapters, the narrative will unfold, encompassing the basics of the sport (Chapter 2), a day at the racetrack (Chapter 3), and the exploration of major races and champions (Chapter 4). Controversies and considerations of animal welfare (Chapter 5), the intricate world of greyhound breeding and bloodlines (Chapter 6), and the key players — owners, trainers, and handlers (Chapter 7) — will all play integral roles in this comprehensive exploration.

In the chapters that follow, we will navigate the business aspects of greyhound racing (Chapter 8), explore its regional influences (Chapter 9), and ponder the future of the sport (Chapter 10). The rise of modern commercial dog racing, a defining chapter in the history of greyhounds, sets the stage for the multifaceted world we are about to uncover, where speed, strategy, and the enduring bond between human and hound converge on the racetrack.

Overview of the Book's Scope and Purpose

As we embark on the pages of "Born to Run - Inside the World of Greyhound Racing," it is essential to grasp the overarching scope and purpose that guides our exploration. This book endeavors to be more than a mere chronicle of greyhound racing; it aims to be a comprehensive journey that uncovers the layers of history, culture, and complexities that define this captivating sport.

The scope of the book is expansive, weaving together the threads of greyhound racing from its ancient origins to the modern-day, encompassing the evolution of the sport on a global scale. It delves into the intricacies of greyhound abilities, their historical roles in societies across different eras, and the transformation of these swift canines from revered companions to competitive athletes.

The narrative unfolds chronologically, beginning with the ancient roots of greyhound racing in Chapter 1. This foundation allows readers to appreciate the gradual transition of greyhounds from symbolic figures in ancient civilizations to the stars of modern racetracks. We traverse through the basics of the sport, experiencing a day at the racetrack, exploring major races and champions, and confronting controversies related to animal welfare.

In Chapter 6, we delve into the world of greyhound breeding and bloodlines, unraveling the science and art behind the creation of exceptional racing dogs. The book introduces readers to the key figures shaping the sport — owners, trainers, and handlers — in Chapter 7, offering insights into their methods, successes, and the profound relationships they share with their canine counterparts.

The business side of greyhound racing takes center stage in Chapter 8, shedding light on the economics, media deals, and regulatory challenges that define the industry. In Chapter 9, we embark on a geographical exploration, tracing the sport's roots in various regions — from the South to the Western US, the Midwest, New England, and the international racing scenes in the UK, Ireland, and Australia.

Chapter 10 peers into the future, examining the shifting public perceptions, legislative changes, and technological advancements that pose both challenges and opportunities for the sport. As we conclude this journey in the final chapter, key takeaways and insights from the world of greyhound racing are reflected upon, and the book's purpose becomes clear: to provide readers with a comprehensive, informative, and nuanced understanding of a sport that goes beyond the racetrack.

The purpose of "Born to Run" is not only to narrate the history of greyhound racing but to foster a connection between the reader and the sport. It aims to ignite a curiosity about the complexities and controversies, the triumphs and challenges, and the enduring bond between humans and greyhounds that define this unique corner of the sporting world.

Through meticulous research, engaging narratives, and a commitment to presenting a balanced view, this book invites readers to step into the world of greyhound racing, where speed meets strategy, and the stories of these remarkable athletes unfold. Whether you are a seasoned enthusiast, a curious observer, or a newcomer to the sport, "Born to Run" aims to be a captivating journey through the history, culture, and future of greyhound racing.

Chapter 1: The Origins of Greyhound Racing
Ancient Roots and Early Appearances in History

To comprehend the origins of greyhound racing, we must embark on a journey through time, tracing the ancient roots and early appearances of these remarkable canines in the annals of history. Long before the modern racetracks and organized competitions, greyhounds held a special place in the hearts of civilizations across the globe.

The tale begins in the sands of ancient Egypt, where greyhounds were not merely dogs but revered companions of pharaohs and symbols of nobility. Hieroglyphics and tomb paintings depict these canines in regal settings, highlighting their grace and loyalty. It was here that the intrinsic connection between humans and greyhounds first flourished, as these swift and elegant creatures became more than mere hunting partners—they became revered members of the royal entourage.

Moving across continents, the ancient Greeks recognized the extraordinary athleticism of greyhounds. In Greek mythology, these canines became associated with the gods, embodying the qualities of swiftness and grace. The Greeks celebrated the prowess of greyhounds not only in the hunting fields but also in the arena of myth, immortalizing them in stories and art.

As the Roman Empire expanded, so did the influence of greyhounds. Romans admired the speed and agility of these dogs, employing them for various tasks, from hunting to guarding estates. Greyhounds were symbols of status and sophistication, finding their place in the grand tapestry of Roman society.

The journey through history takes us to medieval Europe, where greyhounds transitioned from symbols of nobility to indispensable hunting companions. The aristocracy valued these dogs for their speed and keen eyesight, qualities that made them ideal for pursuing game. Paintings from this era capture the regal essence of greyhounds, showcasing them in the company of kings and queens as esteemed members of the royal court.

The Renaissance marked a shift in the perception of greyhounds. No longer confined to the elite, these dogs found their way into the homes of the burgeoning middle class. Their roles diversified from hunting to companionship, and the Renaissance saw the emergence of coursing competitions that pitted greyhounds against each other in friendly races, foreshadowing the organized sport that would emerge centuries later.

In this exploration of ancient roots, it becomes clear that greyhounds were more than utilitarian animals—they were revered and celebrated members of society. Their roles evolved from symbolic companions to functional hunters and, eventually, to the stars of racing tracks. The transition from ancient civilizations to the early appearances in history set the stage for the modern era of greyhound racing, a transition we will further uncover in the subsequent chapters of "Born to Run - Inside the World of Greyhound Racing."

Import to America and Early US Racing

As we navigate the historical landscape of greyhound racing, the narrative takes an intriguing turn as these swift canines make their journey across the Atlantic, finding new terrain in America. The importation of greyhounds to the United States marks a pivotal chapter in the evolution of the sport, laying the groundwork for what would become a thriving industry.

The early 20th century saw a surge in interest in greyhounds as more individuals recognized the potential of these dogs as not just hunting companions but as athletes capable of remarkable speed. It was during this period that greyhounds, often brought by immigrants from Europe, found themselves on American soil, setting the stage for the emergence of organized racing.

Informal races among dog owners became a common sight in open fields, reflecting the innate desire for competition and the thrill of witnessing these canines in action. These impromptu events showcased the natural speed and agility of greyhounds, capturing the imagination of those who witnessed their sprints.

The first organized greyhound races in the United States were grassroots affairs, held on makeshift tracks where enthusiasts gathered to watch these dogs unleash their remarkable abilities. The sport began to take on a more structured form as dedicated individuals recognized the potential for organized events that could cater to a growing audience hungry for entertainment.

As the popularity of greyhound racing began to rise, the need for formalized tracks became evident. In the early stages, these tracks were relatively simple, often no more than dirt paths with minimal infrastructure. However, they marked a departure from the informal races of the past, providing a regulated environment for competitions and enhancing the overall spectator experience.

Professional kennels emerged to meet the demand for well-trained and competitive racing greyhounds. Skilled trainers and handlers, drawing inspiration from the methods employed in other competitive sports, began to refine the techniques and strategies used to prepare these dogs for the rigors of the racetrack.

The establishment of organized tracks and professional kennels laid the foundation for the commercialization of greyhound racing in the United States. The sport, once an informal pastime, was evolving into a legitimate form of entertainment, capturing the attention of a broad audience.

This period of import and early racing in the United States is a testament to the adaptability of greyhounds and the human fascination with their extraordinary abilities. The transition from informal contests to organized events reflects a societal shift towards a more structured and regulated approach to the sport, setting the stage for the golden age of greyhound racing that would soon follow.

As we delve deeper into the origins of greyhound racing, the narrative will unfold in subsequent chapters, exploring the spread of popularity across post-war America, the golden age of the sport, and the establishment of greyhound racing as a cultural phenomenon. The journey through time continues, offering insights into the evolution of a sport that began with informal races on open fields and transformed into the thrilling and organized spectacle we recognize today.

Emergence of Organized Tracks and Professional Kennels

The evolution of greyhound racing in the United States took a significant leap forward with the emergence of organized tracks and the establishment of professional kennels. This transformative period, often regarded as the cornerstone of the sport's development, saw the transition from informal contests to a regulated and commercialized industry.

As the popularity of greyhound racing grew in the early 20th century, the need for more structured and regulated venues became apparent. Informal races held in open fields gave way to purpose-built tracks that could accommodate the burgeoning audience and provide a standardized environment for competitions. The establishment of these tracks marked a turning point, elevating greyhound racing from a local pastime to a formalized and organized sport.

These early tracks were modest in comparison to the modern facilities we recognize today. Often laid out on dirt or grass, they represented a departure from the ad-hoc nature of previous races. These tracks, while basic, provided a platform for the sport to flourish, offering spectators a designated space to witness the grace and speed of racing greyhounds.

Simultaneously, the emergence of professional kennels became integral to the development of greyhound racing. As the demand for competitive and well-trained racing greyhounds increased, skilled trainers and handlers stepped into the spotlight. These professionals brought expertise from other competitive sports, adapting training regimens to enhance the performance of their canine athletes.

Professional kennels not only contributed to the physical conditioning of racing greyhounds but also played a vital role in refining racing strategies. The art of training these dogs to follow a mechanical lure, pacing themselves for optimal speed, became a science that evolved with each generation of trainers. The symbiotic relationship between greyhounds and their human handlers was cemented during this period, laying the foundation for the intricate partnership that defines the sport today.

The establishment of organized tracks and professional kennels had a profound impact on the overall experience of greyhound racing. Spectators were no longer witnessing sporadic races in open spaces; instead, they found themselves immersed in a more regulated and spectator-friendly environment. The transition from informal events to organized races laid the groundwork for the commercialization of greyhound racing, attracting a broader audience and solidifying the sport's status as a legitimate form of entertainment.

Chapter 1, which explores the origins of greyhound racing, now unravels the layers of this critical juncture — the emergence of organized tracks and professional kennels. The narrative continues to unfold in subsequent chapters, tracing the sport's journey through post-war America, the golden age of greyhound racing, and the establishment of greyhound racing as a cultural phenomenon. The story of greyhound racing, born from humble beginnings, gains momentum as it hurtles toward the electrifying spectacle that captivates audiences around the world.

Spread of Popularity Across Post-War America

In the wake of World War II, a wave of change swept across America, and within this transformative period, greyhound racing found fertile ground for unprecedented growth. The post-war era witnessed the sport transcending regional boundaries, capturing the hearts and imaginations of a nation hungry for entertainment and excitement.

As the country emerged from the challenges of war, a sense of optimism and a desire for leisure and recreation took hold. Greyhound racing, with its blend of speed, strategy, and the innate grace of these athletic dogs, provided a perfect outlet for those seeking diversion and amusement. Tracks that had once been confined to specific regions began to multiply, appearing in urban centers and suburban landscapes alike.

The spread of greyhound racing was not merely geographical; it permeated the cultural fabric of post-war America. Tracks became gathering places, social hubs where communities converged to witness the thrilling spectacle of racing greyhounds. Families, friends, and individuals of all backgrounds found themselves drawn to the electrifying atmosphere, marking the sport's transition from a niche activity to a mainstream form of entertainment.

The post-war era also saw advancements in technology, and this played a role in the dissemination of greyhound racing across the nation. The sport, once confined to live events, became increasingly accessible through various media channels. Radio broadcasts and later television coverage brought the excitement of the racetrack into living rooms, allowing a broader audience to experience the thrill of greyhound racing without being physically present.

During this period, greyhound racing became intertwined with the American cultural experience. The sport's popularity was not limited to a specific demographic; instead, it resonated across diverse communities. It became a symbol of post-war prosperity, embodying the nation's spirit of resilience and renewal.

The golden age of greyhound racing was marked by iconic tracks that became synonymous with the sport's rise to prominence. From Florida to California, tracks like Hialeah Park, Wonderland Greyhound Park, and Caliente Racetrack became legendary venues, hosting premier events that drew crowds in the tens of thousands.

As greyhound racing soared in popularity, it also became a significant contributor to the economy. The industry generated employment opportunities, from kennel workers to track staff, and attracted investments from individuals who saw the potential for financial gain. The economic impact of greyhound racing was felt not only at the local level but also at the state and national levels, solidifying its status as a significant industry.

Chapter 1, tracing the origins of greyhound racing, now reveals the fascinating story of its spread across post-war America. The narrative will continue to unfold in subsequent chapters, exploring the intricacies of the sport's evolution, major races and champions, controversies, and the business aspects that define greyhound racing. The journey through history propels us forward, shedding light on how a sport born from humble beginnings captivated the nation and laid the foundation for the vibrant and dynamic world of greyhound racing we know today.

Greyhound Racing's Golden Age

The mid-20th century marked the zenith of greyhound racing's popularity in the United States, a period often referred to as the sport's "Golden Age." As post-war America embraced leisure and entertainment, greyhound racing emerged as a cultural phenomenon, capturing the imagination of a nation and leaving an indelible mark on the history of the sport.

The golden age was characterized by a proliferation of tracks across the country, each vying for attention with grandeur and spectacle. Iconic venues, from the East Coast to the West, became synonymous with the thrill of the racetrack. These tracks were not merely sporting arenas; they were vibrant social spaces, where communities gathered to witness the grace and speed of racing greyhounds.

Hialeah Park in Florida, with its art deco architecture and lush surroundings, became a symbol of glamour and sophistication. Wonderland Greyhound Park in Massachusetts drew crowds with its state-of-the-art facilities and innovative promotions. Caliente Racetrack in Tijuana, Mexico, captured the essence of international competition, drawing visitors from both sides of the border. These and other tracks became stages for the stars of the sport, both canine and human, to showcase their talents.

The golden age was not only marked by the expansion of tracks but also by the emergence of legendary greyhounds that etched their names into the annals of racing history. Names like Mick the Miller, a British greyhound who became a household name in the U.S., and Ballyregan Bob, a prolific racer in the 1980s, became synonymous with excellence on the racetrack.

Their achievements elevated greyhound racing to new heights, captivating audiences and creating lasting legacies.

Major races during this era, such as the Greyhound Derby in the UK and the American Greyhound Derby, became premier events that attracted national attention. The intensity of competition and the pursuit of coveted titles added an extra layer of excitement to the sport. These races became cultural phenomena, drawing spectators from far and wide and contributing to the aura of the golden age.

Beyond the tracks and competitions, greyhound racing permeated popular culture. The sport found its way into literature, film, and art, reflecting its cultural significance. Greyhounds became symbols of speed and elegance, embodying the spirit of an era that valued both athleticism and grace.

The golden age also witnessed advancements in technology that further propelled the sport into the public consciousness. Television broadcasts brought the excitement of the racetrack directly into people's homes, expanding the audience and solidifying greyhound racing as a mainstream form of entertainment.

However, as the sport reached its pinnacle of popularity, it also faced challenges. Controversies, concerns about animal welfare, and changing attitudes toward gambling began to cast a shadow over greyhound racing. The golden age, while glorious, was not immune to the evolving dynamics of societal values and ethical considerations.

Chapter 1, tracing the origins of greyhound racing, now unfolds the captivating story of its golden age. The narrative will continue to evolve in subsequent chapters, exploring the complexities of the sport's history, major races and champions, controversies, and the business aspects that define greyhound racing. The golden age, a chapter of exuberance and accomplishment, sets the stage for the nuanced and dynamic journey through the world of greyhound racing.

Chapter 2: The Basics of the Sport
Types of Races and Track Configurations

In the intricate world of greyhound racing, the sport unfolds on a canvas of various race formats and track configurations. Understanding the nuances of these elements is essential to appreciating the diversity and excitement that defines each competition.

Types of Races:

1. Sprint Races: Sprint races are the heart-pounding, fast-paced contests that showcase the sheer speed of greyhounds. Typically covering distances of 300 to 550 yards, these races are a test of quick acceleration and rapid pacing. Sprint races are exhilarating for both spectators and participants, as greyhounds unleash their remarkable speed over short distances.

2. Route Races: In contrast to sprints, route races challenge greyhounds to cover longer distances, often ranging from 600 to 1,000 yards. These races demand a different set of skills, requiring endurance and strategic pacing. Greyhounds that excel in route races demonstrate a balance of speed and stamina, making these competitions a captivating display of athletic prowess.

3. Hurdle Races: Hurdle races add an extra layer of challenge to the traditional sprint format. Greyhounds navigate obstacles, usually hurdles or jumps, adding an element of strategy and agility to the race. Hurdle races are not as common as sprints or route races but provide a unique spectacle for enthusiasts who appreciate the athleticism and dexterity of racing greyhounds.

4. Handicap Races: Handicap races aim to level the playing field by assigning weights based on the greyhound's past performance. This format allows dogs of varying abilities to compete more evenly. The weights are adjusted to give each greyhound an equal chance of winning, creating an element of unpredictability and excitement for spectators.

Track Configurations:

1. Oval Tracks: The majority of greyhound races take place on oval tracks. These tracks can vary in size, with dimensions influencing the dynamics of the race. Oval tracks are designed to accommodate both sprint and route races, providing versatility for different race formats.

2. Straight Tracks: Less common but equally thrilling, straight tracks offer a unique racing experience. Greyhounds compete in a straight line, usually covering a shorter distance. The absence of turns places a premium on quick acceleration and raw speed, making straight tracks a favorite for spectators who relish rapid-paced contests.

3. Inside and Outside Boxes: The starting boxes, from which greyhounds begin the race, are positioned either on the inside or outside of the track. The choice of box placement can influence a greyhound's strategy, as inside boxes provide a shorter path around the first turn, while outside boxes offer a clearer view of the track. The starting box position adds an additional layer of complexity to the race dynamics.

4. Crossover Tracks: Crossover tracks, featuring a figure-eight or crossover design, add a unique dimension to greyhound racing. Greyhounds navigate a track that intersects with itself, requiring precision and adaptability. Crossover

tracks are less common but offer a distinctive and visually striking racing experience.

Understanding the intricacies of race types and track configurations enhances the appreciation for the sport of greyhound racing. Each element contributes to the multifaceted nature of competitions, where speed, strategy, and the unique qualities of each greyhound converge on the track. As we delve deeper into "The Basics of the Sport," the narrative will continue to unravel, exploring the attributes of successful racing greyhounds, training regimens, racing strategies, and the rules and regulations that govern this thrilling sport.

Attributes of Successful Racing Greyhounds

The world of greyhound racing is a realm where athleticism, instinct, and a unique set of attributes converge to create exceptional athletes. Racing greyhounds, renowned for their speed and agility, possess a combination of physical and temperamental traits that set them apart in the competitive arena. Understanding the attributes that define successful racing greyhounds provides insight into the intricacies of the sport.

1. Speed: At the core of a successful racing greyhound is an innate speed that sets them apart from other dog breeds. Greyhounds are one of the fastest dog breeds, capable of reaching speeds of up to 45 miles per hour. This extraordinary speed is a result of their slender build, powerful hindquarters, and a unique double suspension gallop that propels them forward with exceptional velocity.

2. Agility: Beyond straight-line speed, agility is a crucial attribute for racing greyhounds. Tracks often feature turns and curves, demanding a high degree of maneuverability. Successful greyhounds exhibit nimble footwork, allowing them to navigate the twists and turns of the track with grace and precision. Their agility is a product of well-coordinated movements and a finely tuned sense of balance.

3. Endurance: While speed is paramount in sprint races, endurance becomes a critical factor in longer route races. Successful racing greyhounds possess the stamina to maintain their pace over extended distances. Endurance is a testament to their cardiovascular fitness and the efficiency of their oxygen

utilization, allowing them to sustain peak performance throughout the race.

4. Muscle Tone: Well-defined muscle tone is a visual marker of a healthy and fit racing greyhound. The sleek and muscular physique of these dogs contributes to their power and speed. Their lean build minimizes unnecessary weight, ensuring an optimal power-to-weight ratio that enhances their ability to accelerate and maintain speed.

5. Focus and Determination: Racing greyhounds display an impressive level of focus and determination when on the track. The ability to concentrate on the mechanical lure, navigate the racecourse, and maintain a competitive spirit sets successful greyhounds apart. Their intense focus is a product of training, genetics, and the unique bond they form with their handlers.

6. Temperament: The temperament of a racing greyhound is a delicate balance of competitiveness and sociability. While they exhibit a fierce drive to win on the track, they are known for their gentle and affable nature off the track. This temperament makes them trainable and adaptable to the routines and demands of the racing environment.

7. Intelligence: Racing greyhounds display a level of intelligence that contributes to their ability to learn and execute racing strategies. Intelligent dogs are more responsive to training, enabling handlers to shape their behavior on the track. This intelligence is evident in their capacity to understand commands, follow racing tactics, and adapt to various race conditions.

8. Good Health and Resilience: Maintaining good health is fundamental to a racing greyhound's success. A resilient and robust constitution is essential for withstanding the physical demands of training and racing. Regular veterinary care, a balanced diet, and a supportive training regimen contribute to their overall well-being.

As we delve into the attributes of successful racing greyhounds, it becomes evident that these dogs are finely tuned athletes with a unique combination of physical prowess and mental acuity. The narrative will continue to unfold in subsequent chapters, exploring the training regimens, racing strategies, and the rules and regulations that govern the dynamic world of greyhound racing.

Training Regimens and Exercise Routines

The prowess of a racing greyhound on the track is not solely a result of innate abilities; it is a product of meticulous training regimens and purposeful exercise routines. The journey from a promising pup to a top-tier racing athlete involves a combination of physical conditioning, mental stimulation, and a unique partnership between the greyhound and its handler. Understanding the intricacies of training and exercise unveils the dedication and expertise that go into preparing these remarkable dogs for the rigors of the racetrack.

1. Puppyhood Development: Training begins early in a greyhound's life, often during the puppyhood stage. Handlers focus on socialization, introducing the pups to various environments, sounds, and stimuli. Positive reinforcement techniques are employed to foster a strong bond between the greyhound and its handler, establishing a foundation of trust that will be crucial in later stages of training.

2. Basic Obedience Training: As greyhounds mature, basic obedience training becomes a cornerstone of their development. Handlers teach essential commands such as sit, stay, and recall. These commands lay the groundwork for effective communication between the greyhound and its handler both on and off the track.

3. Track Familiarization: Introducing greyhounds to the racetrack environment is a gradual process. Puppies are exposed to the sights and sounds of the track, helping them acclimate to the unique surroundings. Handlers use positive reinforcement to associate the track with a positive experience, building the greyhound's confidence and curiosity.

4. Mechanical Lure Training: Central to greyhound racing is the pursuit of a mechanical lure. Training involves familiarizing the greyhound with the lure's movement and sound. Initially, the lure is moved at a slower pace, gradually increasing speed as the greyhound becomes more adept. This training enhances the greyhound's prey drive and racing instincts.

5. Physical Conditioning: Greyhounds undergo rigorous physical conditioning to build strength and endurance. Exercise routines include sprinting, interval training, and long-distance running. Treadmills are often used to simulate race conditions, allowing greyhounds to maintain peak fitness levels. Swimming is also incorporated to provide low-impact cardiovascular exercise.

6. Group Training Sessions: Greyhounds thrive on social interaction, and group training sessions contribute to their overall development. These sessions allow greyhounds to run alongside their peers, promoting healthy competition and camaraderie. Group training not only enhances physical fitness but also sharpens racing instincts as greyhounds learn to navigate the track in the presence of other dogs.

7. Nutritional Care: A balanced and nutritious diet is a fundamental aspect of a greyhound's training regimen. Handlers work closely with veterinarians and nutritionists to ensure that greyhounds receive the optimal combination of proteins, fats, and carbohydrates. Nutritional care is tailored to the individual needs of each greyhound based on factors such as age, health, and activity level.

8. Rest and Recovery: Adequate rest and recovery are integral to a greyhound's overall well-being. Training schedules include designated rest days to prevent overexertion and reduce the risk of injuries. Handlers monitor each greyhound's condition closely, adjusting training intensity based on individual responses to ensure sustained peak performance.

9. Mental Stimulation: Mental stimulation is as vital as physical exercise in a greyhound's training routine. Puzzle toys, interactive games, and novel experiences keep their minds sharp and engaged. Mental stimulation contributes to a well-balanced and content racing greyhound, fostering a positive attitude toward training and racing.

10. Continuous Assessment and Adaptation: Training regimens are dynamic and subject to continuous assessment. Handlers closely monitor each greyhound's progress, adjusting training plans as needed. Individualized approaches consider factors such as temperament, response to training, and any signs of stress or fatigue.

Training regimens and exercise routines are a harmonious blend of science, art, and intuition. The bond between greyhound and handler is a symbiotic relationship, where mutual understanding and trust form the bedrock of success. As we continue our exploration of "The Basics of the Sport," subsequent chapters will delve into the racing strategies, rules, and regulations that further define the world of greyhound racing.

Racing Strategies and Techniques

At the intersection of skill, speed, and instinct, racing strategies and techniques come to the forefront in the dynamic world of greyhound racing. A successful race is not solely about raw speed but also involves a carefully orchestrated dance of tactics, with each greyhound and handler pairing bringing its unique approach to the track. Understanding the intricacies of racing strategies unveils the artistry and nuance that define each competition.

1. Box Break and Acceleration: The opening moments of a race, known as the box break, set the tone for the entire competition. Greyhounds burst from starting boxes with explosive acceleration. Racing strategies often hinge on a greyhound's ability to make a swift and clean break, gaining an early advantage over competitors. Handlers work on refining a greyhound's starting technique to maximize speed from the outset.

2. Positioning and Racing Lines: Greyhound racing is not a simple sprint but a strategic navigation of the track. Handlers train greyhounds to adopt optimal racing lines, taking turns efficiently and minimizing the distance traveled. Strategic positioning during the race is crucial, and handlers may employ tactics such as hugging the rail or taking wider turns based on their greyhound's strengths and the dynamics of the competition.

3. Pacing and Energy Conservation: Understanding the pacing of a race is essential for conserving energy over the course. Greyhounds are trained to find a balance between maintaining a competitive speed and conserving energy for the

final stretch. Handlers often employ interval training techniques to enhance a greyhound's ability to regulate its pace and reserve energy for crucial moments in the race.

4. Drafting and Strategic Positioning: Similar to other racing sports, greyhound racing involves elements of drafting. Greyhounds may strategically position themselves behind a competitor, using the leading dog to break the wind resistance. This drafting technique can conserve energy, providing an opportunity for a well-timed surge toward the finish line.

5. Reading the Mechanical Lure: The mechanical lure, a pivotal element in greyhound racing, requires a keen understanding from both greyhound and handler. Racing strategies involve training greyhounds to focus on the lure, anticipating its movements and responding with precision. Handlers may employ techniques to enhance a greyhound's ability to track the lure effectively, ensuring an optimal racing experience.

6. Adaptability to Track Conditions: Track conditions can vary, influencing the effectiveness of different racing strategies. A wet track may require adjustments in pacing and turns, while a dry and firm surface may favor certain greyhounds with specific running styles. Handlers assess track conditions and tailor training regimens to enhance a greyhound's adaptability to different racing environments.

7. Tactical Use of Strengths: Greyhounds, like athletes in any sport, have individual strengths and weaknesses. Racing strategies involve identifying and leveraging a greyhound's strengths during a race. Some greyhounds may excel in acceleration, while others may possess exceptional endurance.

Handlers tailor racing strategies to amplify their greyhound's unique attributes for a competitive edge.

8. Training for Race Distances: The length of a race significantly influences racing strategies. Greyhounds are trained for specific race distances, and handlers adjust their strategies accordingly. Sprint races demand explosive bursts of speed, while route races require a combination of speed and endurance. Tailoring training for specific race distances optimizes a greyhound's performance on the track.

9. Finish Line Tactics: The final stretch of a race often determines the outcome. Racing strategies for the finish line involve ensuring that a greyhound has the energy reserves for a powerful sprint. Handlers may employ drills that simulate the closing moments of a race, fine-tuning a greyhound's ability to surge ahead and secure victory as they approach the finish line.

10. Post-Race Recovery and Analysis: Racing strategies extend beyond the track to the post-race phase. Handlers carefully observe their greyhound's recovery, analyzing the race's dynamics and identifying areas for improvement. Post-race recovery includes cooldown exercises, proper hydration, and attentive care to ensure the greyhound is in optimal condition for subsequent competitions.

Racing strategies and techniques are a blend of science, observation, and the unique connection between greyhound and handler. The symbiotic relationship forged through training and competition shapes the strategies employed on the track. As we continue our exploration of "The Basics of the Sport," subsequent chapters will delve into the rules and regulations, major races, controversies, and the business aspects that contribute to the rich tapestry of greyhound racing.

Rules and Regulations of Races

Greyhound racing, like any organized sport, operates within a framework of rules and regulations designed to ensure fair competition, the well-being of the dogs, and the integrity of the races. Understanding these rules provides insight into the structure and ethical considerations that govern the world of greyhound racing.

1. Starting Procedures: Races commence with a standardized starting procedure. Greyhounds are loaded into starting boxes, typically positioned along the track's inner rail. Once secured, the starting boxes open simultaneously, releasing the greyhounds onto the track. The simultaneous release ensures fair competition, and strict protocols are in place to address any irregularities during the starting process.

2. Track Dimensions: Greyhound tracks adhere to specific dimensions to maintain consistency across races. The length of the track varies depending on the race type, with sprint tracks typically shorter than those designed for route races. The width of the track is also standardized, ensuring a level playing field for all competitors.

3. Mechanical Lure Operation: The mechanical lure, a key component of greyhound racing, follows a predetermined course to entice the greyhounds. The lure's speed and movements are carefully regulated to simulate prey and maintain the excitement of the chase. Rules dictate the proper operation of the lure, preventing deviations that could unfairly advantage or disadvantage specific greyhounds.

4. Race Distances and Categories: Greyhound races are categorized based on distance, with distinct rules for sprint and

route races. Sprint races typically cover shorter distances, while route races involve longer courses. Each category has its own set of regulations, ensuring that greyhounds are appropriately trained and conditioned for the specific demands of their race.

5. Weight Distribution: Handicap races involve assigning weights to greyhounds based on their past performances. The goal is to create a more balanced competition, allowing dogs of varying abilities to compete on a level playing field. The weights are carefully calculated to account for a greyhound's racing history and recent performances.

6. Racing Attire: Greyhounds race without traditional collars to prevent injury during competition. Instead, they wear racing blankets, which serve both as identification and a way to minimize the risk of entanglement. Racing blankets are color-coded to represent the greyhound's starting position and facilitate clear identification during the race.

7. Judges and Race Calls: Judges oversee each race, ensuring that all rules are followed and adjudicating any infractions. They monitor the start, progression, and finish of each race, and their decisions are final. Race calls, conducted by experienced announcers, provide real-time commentary to spectators, enhancing the overall viewing experience.

8. Doping Control: To maintain the integrity of the sport, strict anti-doping measures are in place. Greyhounds are subject to random drug testing, and substances that could enhance performance or compromise the health of the dogs are strictly prohibited. Doping control is a crucial component of ensuring fair and ethical competition.

9. Injuries and Veterinary Care: In the event of injuries during a race, veterinary care is promptly provided. The welfare of the greyhounds is paramount, and any injured dog receives immediate attention. Races may be stopped if safety concerns arise, and injured greyhounds are carefully assessed and treated to ensure their well-being.

10. Retirement and Adoption: Rules are in place to address the post-racing phase of a greyhound's career. When a greyhound retires from racing, responsible rehoming and adoption programs are encouraged. Many racing organizations collaborate with adoption agencies to ensure that retired greyhounds find loving homes, marking the end of their competitive careers on a positive note.

Understanding and adhering to these rules and regulations is essential for all stakeholders in the greyhound racing community. The framework ensures a level playing field, safeguards the welfare of the dogs, and upholds the ethical standards that define the sport. As we progress through subsequent chapters, the exploration will continue, delving into major races, controversies, the business of greyhound racing, and the sport's diverse regional influences.

Chapter 3: A Day at the Racetrack
Arriving at the Track and Reading the Program

The anticipation builds as spectators, enthusiasts, and participants converge on the greyhound racetrack for a day filled with excitement, competition, and the thrill of the chase. Arriving at the track is not just a physical journey; it marks the beginning of an immersive experience that combines the social, strategic, and adrenaline-fueled aspects of greyhound racing.

Arrival and Atmosphere:

1. Early Enthusiasts: Devoted fans and enthusiasts often arrive early, eager to secure prime seating and soak in the atmosphere. The early hours are filled with a sense of camaraderie as attendees share their passion for the sport, exchange insights, and engage in friendly banter.

2. Entrance and Ticketing: Arriving spectators make their way through the entrance gates, where ticketing and security procedures are seamlessly managed. The ticketing process allows attendees to choose from various seating options, ranging from general admission areas to premium grandstands, enhancing the overall experience.

3. Trackside Ambiance: The trackside ambiance is a unique blend of excitement and anticipation. The air is filled with the sounds of distant barking, the murmur of conversations, and the occasional cheer from early winners at the betting windows. The scent of concession stands adds to the sensory tapestry, creating an unmistakable racetrack atmosphere.

Reading the Program:

1. Program Distribution: Before diving into the races, attendees acquire the essential guide to the day's events—the racing program. These programs, available at various points around the track, provide a comprehensive overview of the greyhounds, their past performances, and the race schedule.

2. Race Schedule and Start Times: The program meticulously details the race schedule, including start times for each event. Spectators consult the schedule to plan their day, ensuring they don't miss the races they are most eager to watch. The anticipation builds as the first race approaches, and attendees gather near the track, eagerly awaiting the spectacle.

3. Greyhound Lineup: Each race features a lineup of greyhounds, and the program introduces these canine athletes to the audience. Details such as the greyhound's name, racing history, and recent performances are outlined, allowing spectators to assess the contenders and make informed decisions when placing bets.

4. Statistics and Performance Data: In-depth statistics and performance data are key components of the racing program. Attendees pore over these details, analyzing a greyhound's recent form, average race times, and preferred racing style. The program serves as a valuable tool for both seasoned bettors and newcomers, guiding them in making informed wagers.

5. Trainer and Handler Information: The racing program doesn't just focus on the greyhounds; it also sheds light on the trainers and handlers. Attendees learn about the individuals behind the scenes, their strategies, and past successes. This information adds a personal touch to the racing

experience, fostering connections between the audience and the key figures in the sport.

6. Race Conditions and Track Information: The program provides crucial details about race conditions and the state of the track. Factors such as weather conditions, track surface, and potential influences on race outcomes are outlined. Attendees factor in this information when assessing the greyhounds' ability to perform under specific conditions.

7. Betting Odds and Payouts: Betting odds and potential payouts are prominently featured in the program. Attendees study these odds, considering factors such as recent performances, track conditions, and the greyhound's racing style. The dynamic odds add an additional layer of excitement as spectators make their selections and place bets.

8. Educational Resources: Racing programs often include educational resources to enhance the understanding of the sport. Glossaries of racing terms, explanations of betting types, and insights into greyhound anatomy and behavior serve as valuable resources for both novices and seasoned enthusiasts.

As attendees absorb the information from the racing program, the excitement builds, setting the stage for the heart-pounding moments that lie ahead. Armed with knowledge and fueled by anticipation, spectators are ready to immerse themselves in the world of greyhound racing, where every race is a unique spectacle, and every greyhound has the potential to become a champion.

Wagering - How to Bet on the Dogs

At the heart of the greyhound racing experience lies the exhilarating world of wagering. The racetrack transforms into a buzzing arena of anticipation and strategic decision-making as spectators engage in the age-old tradition of betting on their chosen greyhounds. Understanding the nuances of wagering adds a layer of excitement and involvement, turning each race into a thrilling opportunity for spectators to test their instincts and, with a bit of luck, reap the rewards.

Introduction to Wagering:

1. Betting as Tradition: Wagering on greyhound races is deeply ingrained in the sport's culture. From seasoned gamblers to casual spectators, the racetrack offers a diverse range of betting options, allowing individuals to participate at their comfort level. The allure of potentially turning a small investment into a substantial payout captivates both seasoned enthusiasts and newcomers.

2. Betting Windows and Tote Boards: At the racetrack, betting windows are focal points where attendees place their bets. The vibrant display of odds and potential payouts on the tote board captures the attention of the crowd. Attendees study the information provided, assessing the odds and making informed decisions before stepping up to the betting windows to place their wagers.

Types of Bets:

1. Win, Place, and Show: The simplest and most common forms of bets are Win, Place, and Show.

- A Win bet is a wager on a specific greyhound to finish first.

- A Place bet is a wager on a greyhound to finish either first or second.

- A Show bet is a wager on a greyhound to finish in the top three.

2. Across the Board: The Across the Board bet combines Win, Place, and Show into a single wager. If the chosen greyhound wins, the bettor receives payouts for all three positions. If the greyhound places or shows, corresponding payouts are still awarded.

3. Quinella: A Quinella bet involves selecting two greyhounds to finish first and second in any order. This bet adds an element of flexibility, allowing bettors to win as long as their chosen greyhounds occupy the top two positions.

4. Exacta: The Exacta bet is more specific, requiring bettors to predict the exact order of the first and second-place finishers. This bet offers higher payouts due to its increased level of difficulty.

5. Trifecta: For those seeking an even greater challenge, the Trifecta bet involves selecting the first, second, and third-place finishers in the correct order. While difficult, successful Trifecta bets yield substantial payouts.

6. Superfecta: The Superfecta bet takes it a step further, requiring bettors to predict the first four finishers in the correct order. This bet is challenging but offers lucrative rewards for those who accurately forecast the race outcome.

Factors Influencing Betting Decisions:

1. Greyhound Form and Performance: Studying a greyhound's recent form and performance is crucial for making informed betting decisions. Factors such as past race results,

average times, and racing style contribute to assessing a greyhound's potential in the current race.

2. Track Conditions: The state of the track, including factors like weather and surface conditions, plays a significant role in betting. Some greyhounds may perform better on wet tracks, while others excel on dry surfaces. Bettors factor in these conditions when making their selections.

3. Trainer and Handler Influence: The reputation and track record of a greyhound's trainer and handler are important considerations. Successful trainers and handlers often have a keen understanding of the sport, influencing a greyhound's training, preparation, and race-day performance.

4. Odds and Payouts: The odds displayed on the tote board guide betting decisions. Understanding how odds translate to potential payouts is essential. While lower odds indicate a favored greyhound, higher odds suggest an underdog with the potential for a higher payout.

5. Race Distance: Different greyhounds may excel at specific race distances. Bettors consider the length of the race and how well a greyhound's past performances align with the current race conditions.

6. Intuition and Gut Feeling: Betting on greyhounds isn't solely a science; it's also an art. Some bettors rely on intuition, gut feelings, or a connection with a particular greyhound to guide their decisions. This subjective element adds an element of unpredictability to the betting experience.

Placing a Wager:

1. Selecting a Betting Type: Bettors begin by selecting the type of bet they wish to place. Novices often start with

simpler bets like Win, Place, or Show, while more experienced bettors may explore Exacta, Trifecta, or Superfecta options.

2. Choosing Greyhounds: With the betting type in mind, bettors choose the greyhound(s) they believe will perform well in the race. Factors such as recent form, track conditions, and odds influence these decisions.

3. Approaching the Betting Windows: Bettors approach the betting windows with their selections and chosen betting type in hand. Attendants assist in processing bets, providing information on odds, potential payouts, and ensuring that wagers are accurately recorded.

4. Placing the Bet: Bettors confirm their selections, the chosen betting type, and the amount they wish to wager. Once confirmed, the attendant processes the bet, and a ticket is issued as a record of the wager.

5. Watching the Race: With bets placed, spectators eagerly watch the race unfold. The roar of the crowd intensifies as the greyhounds dash toward the finish line, and the outcome determines the success of each wager.

Collecting Winnings:

1. Winning Tickets: Bettors holding winning tickets eagerly proceed to the payout windows. Each type of bet has a designated payout, and attendants calculate the winnings based on the odds and amount wagered.

2. Payout Process: Payouts are efficiently processed, with attendants verifying winning tickets and dispensing cash or vouchers. The thrill of collecting winnings adds to the overall satisfaction of a successful bet.

3. Reflecting on the Experience: Whether celebrating a successful wager or reflecting on the unpredictable nature of greyhound racing, attendees carry the experience with them. The camaraderie, the excitement of the races, and the strategic decision-making contribute to the lasting appeal of wagering on greyhound races.

Responsible Betting Practices:

1. Setting Limits: Responsible betting involves setting limits on the amount of money one is willing to wager. Establishing a budget ensures that betting remains an enjoyable and controlled activity.

2. Understanding Risks: Bettors should be aware of the inherent risks in gambling. While winning is exhilarating, losses are also part of the experience. Understanding the risks helps maintain a balanced and healthy approach to betting.

3. Enjoying the Experience: Wagering on greyhound races is not solely about financial gain; it's an integral part of the overall racing experience. Enjoying the thrill of the races, engaging with fellow enthusiasts, and appreciating the athleticism of the greyhounds contribute to a well-rounded and fulfilling day at the racetrack.

In conclusion, wagering on greyhound races adds an interactive and dynamic dimension to the spectator experience. Whether placing a straightforward Win bet or delving into the intricacies of exotic bets like Trifecta and Superfecta, each wager represents a unique opportunity to engage with the sport and, for a moment, become part of the drama that unfolds on the track. As we delve deeper into the world of greyhound racing in subsequent chapters, we will explore behind-the-scenes aspects, major races, controversies, and the multifaceted business of this fascinating sport.

Pregame Rituals and Trackside Traditions

Before the first greyhound takes off from the starting boxes, a day at the racetrack is enveloped in a tapestry of pregame rituals and trackside traditions. These cherished customs not only enhance the overall experience for attendees but also contribute to the unique culture and sense of community that defines greyhound racing venues across the globe. From the early morning preparations to the post-race celebrations, each ritual and tradition adds a layer of richness to the tapestry of the racetrack experience.

Morning Preparations and Kennel Visits:

1. Sunrise at the Track: The day at the racetrack begins with the soft glow of sunrise, casting a warm hue on the track. Enthusiasts and early birds alike embrace the quiet moments before the rush, savoring the serenity of the track awakening to a day of racing.

2. Stable Tours and Kennel Visits: For those eager to delve into the behind-the-scenes world of greyhound racing, stable tours and kennel visits are a must. Attendees have the opportunity to witness the morning routines, observe the care and attention given to the greyhounds, and gain insights into the daily lives of these remarkable athletes.

3. Morning Workouts: As the sun climbs higher, the track comes alive with the rhythmic sound of greyhounds on morning workouts. Trainers guide their charges through practice sprints, fine-tuning their skills and ensuring they are primed for peak performance in upcoming races. Observing these workouts is an immersive prelude to the day's racing spectacle.

Pre-Race Gatherings and Camaraderie:

1. Trackside Breakfasts: Many racetracks offer trackside breakfasts, creating a communal atmosphere where attendees can gather, share insights, and fuel up for the day ahead. The smell of freshly brewed coffee mingles with the excitement in the air as spectators prepare for the first race.

2. Discussion Groups and Tip Exchanges: Pregame rituals often include informal discussion groups where attendees exchange tips, insights, and predictions for the upcoming races. These gatherings, whether organized or spontaneous, foster a sense of camaraderie among spectators who share a common passion for greyhound racing.

3. Morning Line Analysis: The morning line, an early set of odds determined by experts, becomes a focal point for pre-race analysis. Attendees study the morning line, assess the odds, and engage in friendly debates about the potential outcomes of each race. This analytical camaraderie enhances the overall enjoyment of the racing experience.

Lucky Charms and Superstitions:

1. Lucky Numbers and Colors: Superstitions abound at the racetrack, with attendees often having lucky numbers, colors, or specific greyhounds that they believe bring good fortune. Whether it's a lucky charm worn as a talisman or a preferred starting box number, these superstitions add a touch of whimsy to the pregame atmosphere.

2. Good Luck Rituals: Some attendees have pre-race rituals they believe bring good luck. From a particular way of placing bets to following a routine for selecting favorite greyhounds, these rituals create a personal connection to the

racing experience and contribute to the overall sense of anticipation.

Betting Window Excitement:

1. Queueing Up at the Betting Windows: As race time approaches, the energy at the betting windows intensifies. Attendees line up to place their bets, exchanging friendly banter and sharing last-minute tips. The hum of excitement builds as each person eagerly awaits their turn to contribute to the collective anticipation.

2. Final Odds Check: Before placing their bets, attendees conduct a final odds check, ensuring they have the latest information on each greyhound's odds and potential payouts. This last-minute assessment adds a strategic element to the betting process, heightening the thrill of decision-making.

Race Day Attire and Fashion:

1. Dressing for the Occasion: Attendees often embrace the opportunity to dress up for a day at the racetrack. While there's no strict dress code, many choose to don their Sunday best or adopt a style that reflects the elegance and tradition associated with horse and greyhound racing events.

2. Hats and Fascinators: The tradition of wearing hats and fascinators, reminiscent of horse racing culture, has found its way to greyhound racing events. Attendees, especially on major race days, showcase a variety of stylish headwear, adding a touch of glamour to the trackside fashion scene.

National Anthems and Pomp:

1. Patriotic Traditions: On special race days, the playing of national anthems is a poignant moment that adds a sense of ceremony to the proceedings. Attendees stand in respectful

observance, expressing pride and unity as the anthems resonate through the racetrack.

2. Parade of Greyhounds: Before the races begin, a parade of greyhounds introduces the competitors to the audience. This ceremonial procession allows attendees to appreciate the beauty and athleticism of the greyhounds up close, creating a festive atmosphere and building anticipation for the upcoming races.

Post-Race Celebrations and Reflections:

1. Victory Celebrations: Post-race celebrations are an integral part of the racetrack experience. Winning owners, trainers, and handlers share the joy with their greyhounds in the winner's circle. Cheers, applause, and sometimes even victory laps contribute to the jubilant atmosphere that follows a successful race.

2. Reflecting on the Day: As the day concludes, attendees often linger, reflecting on the highs and lows of the races. Discussions about memorable moments, surprising upsets, and standout performances create a communal sense of shared experience, fostering a connection among those who have spent the day immersed in the world of greyhound racing.

In essence, the pregame rituals and trackside traditions woven into a day at the racetrack add depth and character to the overall experience. Whether it's the thrill of morning workouts, the camaraderie of breakfast gatherings, or the whimsy of lucky charms, these rituals contribute to the unique fabric of greyhound racing culture. As we continue our exploration of the world of greyhound racing in the subsequent chapters, we'll delve into major races, controversies, the business aspects, and the regional influences that shape this captivating sport.

The culmination of anticipation, strategy, and the thundering paws of racing greyhounds—the race experience is the heartbeat of a day at the racetrack. As spectators gather trackside, the mechanical lure, a whirring mechanism designed to mimic prey, takes center stage, guiding the swift and agile greyhounds on a pursuit that captivates the audience. In this chapter, we delve into the intricacies of the race experience, exploring the dynamics of the chase, the thrill of the finish line, and the unique role played by the mechanical lure.

The Mechanical Lure:

1. Origins and Evolution: The concept of using a mechanical lure to entice greyhounds traces back to the early days of organized racing. What began as a rudimentary system has evolved into a sophisticated apparatus—a motorized device affixed to a track-mounted cable, capable of simulating the unpredictable movements of prey.

2. Lure Operation and Speed: The mechanical lure operates at varying speeds, determined by the type of race and the distance to be covered. As the lure races along the track, greyhounds eagerly pursue, their instincts propelling them forward in a display of breathtaking speed and agility.

3. Pre-Race Lure Inspection: Before each race, a ritualized inspection of the mechanical lure takes place. Handlers and officials ensure that the lure is in optimal condition, free from any irregularities that could affect the race. This meticulous process underscores the commitment to fair and safe competition.

The Chase Unfolds:

1. Starting Box Release: The race begins with the simultaneous release of greyhounds from their starting boxes. The mechanical lure, already in motion, lures the dogs forward, triggering an explosive burst of speed as they accelerate down the track. The sight of sleek and powerful greyhounds in pursuit is a visual spectacle that commands the attention of all present.

2. Chasing the Lure: Greyhounds, driven by their innate hunting instincts, focus intently on the mechanical lure. The chase unfolds with a seamless blend of speed, precision, and anticipation. As the lure speeds ahead, greyhounds engage in a breathtaking pursuit, demonstrating their remarkable athleticism and racing prowess.

3. Strategy and Positioning: Within the race, strategy plays a pivotal role. Greyhounds exhibit different racing styles— some sprint to the front early, while others employ a strategic burst of speed in the final stretch. Observant spectators analyze the dynamics of the chase, noting the positioning of each greyhound and predicting potential shifts in the race's outcome.

Thrills at the Finish Line:

1. Final Stretch Dramatics: As the greyhounds approach the final stretch, the excitement reaches a crescendo. The mechanical lure hurtles toward the finish line, and the greyhounds, spurred on by the lure and the cheers of the crowd, unleash a final burst of speed. The atmosphere is charged with anticipation as spectators root for their chosen contenders.

2. Photo Finishes and Close Calls: Greyhound races often feature photo finishes, moments of suspense where the closeness of the race requires careful examination of photographic evidence to determine the winner. These close

calls add an element of unpredictability, keeping spectators on the edge of their seats until the final results are confirmed.

Behind the Scenes - Life in the Racing Kennels:

1. Post-Race Retrieval: After crossing the finish line, greyhounds slow down, and handlers promptly retrieve them. The immediate post-race moments are crucial for assessing the well-being of the dogs, checking for any signs of fatigue or injury.

2. Cooling Down and Hydration: Handlers guide greyhounds to designated areas for cooling down and hydration. Special attention is given to ensuring the dogs remain in optimal physical condition, with access to water and cooling measures to regulate body temperature.

3. Recovery and Rest: Post-race recovery is a vital aspect of a greyhound's care. Handlers monitor the dogs closely, providing necessary rest and attending to any specific needs. The well-being of the greyhounds is a top priority, and their health and comfort are carefully tended to between races.

Spectator Engagement - Following the Race:

1. Announcer Commentary: The race experience is enhanced by the commentary of skilled announcers who guide spectators through the unfolding drama. Their energetic and insightful commentary provides context, highlights key moments, and elevates the overall enjoyment for those in attendance.

2. Replays and Analysis: Post-race replays and analyses are common features in modern racing venues. Spectators, bettors, and enthusiasts have the opportunity to review the race from multiple angles, gaining a deeper understanding of the

strategies employed, the dynamics of the chase, and the factors influencing the outcome.

The Role of the Crowd:

1. Roar of the Crowd: The crowd plays a pivotal role in the race experience. The roar of the crowd, building as the greyhounds approach the finish line, adds an electric energy to the atmosphere. Spectators become active participants, collectively celebrating triumphs and sharing in the excitement of each race.

2. Collective Exuberance and Disappointment: The collective exuberance of a cheering crowd is matched only by the shared disappointment when favored contenders fall short. The emotional ebb and flow within the crowd create a dynamic backdrop to the races, connecting individuals through their common investment in the outcomes.

Conclusion of the Race:

1. Acknowledging the Winners: As the results are confirmed, winners are acknowledged and celebrated. The presentation of trophies or other accolades adds a ceremonial touch to the proceedings, honoring the achievements of the greyhounds, their handlers, and the connections.

2. Transition to the Next Race: The swift transition from one race to the next is a hallmark of greyhound racing. Attendees, fueled by the energy of the previous race, eagerly turn their attention to the next set of contenders, ready to immerse themselves in the excitement of yet another chase.

In conclusion, the race experience is the heartbeat of a day at the racetrack, weaving together the athleticism of greyhounds, the precision of the mechanical lure, and the collective spirit of the spectators. As we progress through the subsequent chapters, we'll explore major races, controversies, the intricacies of greyhound breeding, and the multifaceted dimensions of the business that sustains this thrilling and enduring sport.

Behind the Scenes - Life in the Racing Kennels

While the racetrack is the stage where the athleticism and speed of greyhounds are on full display, the racing kennels serve as the backstage, where the care, training, and well-being of these remarkable athletes take center stage. In this chapter, we'll venture behind the scenes, exploring the bustling world of the racing kennels, where handlers, trainers, and support staff work in harmony to prepare greyhounds for the thrilling pursuits that await them on the track.

Morning Rituals and Daily Care:

1. Dawn in the Kennels: The day in the racing kennels begins with the first light of dawn. Handlers and trainers arrive early to commence the daily routines that are essential for the health and preparation of the greyhounds. The calm of the early morning provides a serene backdrop for the activities that unfold.

2. Feeding and Nutrition: Proper nutrition is paramount in the life of a racing greyhound. Each greyhound's diet is carefully curated to meet its specific needs, taking into consideration factors such as age, weight, and overall health. High-quality dog food, supplements, and regular feeding schedules contribute to the optimal physical condition of the athletes.

3. Health Checks and Veterinary Care: Regular health checks are conducted to monitor the well-being of the greyhounds. Veterinary professionals play a crucial role in ensuring that the dogs are in prime condition. Vaccinations, dental care, and preventive measures are administered to maintain the health and longevity of these canine athletes.

Training Regimens and Exercise:

1. Morning Workouts: The morning sun witnesses the commencement of training regimens. Handlers, often working in collaboration with trainers, guide the greyhounds through a series of exercises and sprints. The track becomes a dynamic training ground where the dogs hone their racing skills and build the endurance required for competitive pursuits.

2. Swimming and Cross-Training: To diversify training routines and promote overall fitness, some racing kennels incorporate swimming sessions and cross-training exercises. Swimming, in particular, provides a low-impact yet effective workout, enhancing cardiovascular health and muscle strength.

3. Individualized Training Plans: Recognizing that each greyhound is unique, trainers develop individualized training plans. Factors such as racing style, preferred distances, and response to training methods are considered in tailoring regimens that maximize the potential of each dog.

Bonding Between Handlers and Greyhounds:

1. Personal Connections: Handlers forge strong bonds with the greyhounds under their care. This personal connection goes beyond the functional aspects of training and care, creating a relationship built on trust and mutual understanding. Handlers become attuned to the nuances of each dog's personality, preferences, and moods.

2. Comfort and Reassurance: Racing kennels prioritize the comfort and well-being of the greyhounds. Handlers provide reassurance and companionship, helping the dogs feel secure in their environment. This positive interaction extends

to moments of rest and relaxation, contributing to the overall mental and emotional health of the canine athletes.

Post-Training Recovery:

1. Cooling Down and Hydration: After intense training sessions, a meticulous cooling down process ensues. Greyhounds are given ample time to cool down, often in designated areas equipped with shade and cooling mechanisms. Hydration is a priority, with handlers ensuring that each dog has access to fresh water to replenish fluids lost during exercise.

2. Massage and Physiotherapy: Some racing kennels incorporate massage and physiotherapy into the post-training routine. These practices aid in muscle recovery, alleviate tension, and contribute to the overall physical well-being of the greyhounds. Trained professionals work in collaboration with handlers to address specific needs and promote optimal health.

Pre-Race Preparations:

1. Race-Day Rituals: As race day approaches, the racing kennels buzz with heightened activity. Handlers engage in pre-race rituals, preparing the greyhounds both mentally and physically for the upcoming challenges. These rituals may include familiarization with the track, gentle warm-ups, and reinforcing positive associations with the racing experience.

2. Final Health Checks: Before each race, a final round of health checks ensures that the greyhounds are in peak condition. This comprehensive assessment includes a review of vital signs, muscle condition, and overall readiness. Any concerns or signs of fatigue are addressed promptly to prioritize the well-being of the dogs.

Between Races:

1. Rest and Recuperation: Greyhounds, like any athletes, require sufficient rest and downtime between races. Racing kennels provide comfortable sleeping quarters where the dogs can relax and recuperate. Adequate rest is essential for maintaining energy levels and sustaining peak performance throughout a racing season.

2. Socialization and Playtime: Socialization is a key aspect of a greyhound's life in the racing kennels. Handlers facilitate playtime and interactions between the dogs, fostering a sense of camaraderie. These moments of socialization contribute to the overall happiness and contentment of the greyhounds.

Retirement and Adoption Programs:

1. Planning for Retirement: Racing kennels actively plan for the retirement of greyhounds. Handlers and trainers assess each dog's career trajectory and identify an appropriate time for retirement based on factors such as age and performance. This thoughtful approach ensures a smooth transition into post-racing life.

2. Adoption Initiatives: Many racing kennels are involved in adoption programs that facilitate the transition of retired greyhounds to loving homes. These initiatives prioritize the well-being of the dogs beyond their racing careers, promoting responsible ownership and providing opportunities for greyhounds to enjoy a fulfilling life as companions.

Handler Education and Professional Development:

1. Continuous Learning: Handlers undergo continuous education and training to stay abreast of advancements in greyhound care and training methodologies. Workshops,

seminars, and collaborative learning experiences contribute to the ongoing professional development of handlers, ensuring that they provide the best possible care for the greyhounds under their charge.

2. Emphasis on Welfare: Racing kennels place a strong emphasis on the welfare of the greyhounds. This commitment extends beyond the track, encompassing all aspects of the dogs' lives. Handlers are instrumental in championing the welfare of greyhounds, advocating for ethical treatment and the implementation of best practices in the industry.

Conclusion - A Lifelong Commitment:

Life in the racing kennels is a testament to the dedication, expertise, and compassion of handlers and trainers. As we continue our exploration of the world of greyhound racing in subsequent chapters, we'll delve into major races, controversies, the business aspects of the sport, and the regional influences that shape this captivating world. The racing kennels stand as a hub of activity, where the symbiotic relationship between humans and greyhounds unfolds in a tapestry of care, training, and mutual respect.

Chapter 4: Major Races and Champions
The Sport's Classic Races and Prizes

In the illustrious world of greyhound racing, certain events stand out as milestones, showcasing the pinnacle of athleticism, strategy, and competitive spirit. These classic races, steeped in tradition and history, bring together the finest greyhounds, the most skilled trainers, and the enthusiastic roar of spectators. In this chapter, we will explore the sport's classic races and the coveted prizes that have become synonymous with excellence and prestige.

The Derby Classics:

1. The English Greyhound Derby: Founded in 1927, the English Greyhound Derby is one of the oldest and most prestigious races in the world. Run over a distance of 500 meters, this classic event is held annually at Towcester and has a rich legacy of showcasing the best talents in the sport. Greyhounds from around the globe aspire to etch their names in the annals of the English Greyhound Derby's storied history.

2. The Irish Greyhound Derby: The Irish Greyhound Derby, inaugurated in 1928, holds a special place in the hearts of greyhound enthusiasts. Taking place at Shelbourne Park in Dublin, this race attracts top-tier competitors from Ireland and beyond. The dynamic atmosphere and the track's unique challenges contribute to the allure of the Irish Greyhound Derby.

3. The Scottish Greyhound Derby: While not as ancient as its English and Irish counterparts, the Scottish Greyhound Derby, established in 1928, has earned its reputation as a distinguished event. Shawfield Stadium in Glasgow serves as

the venue for this thrilling race, offering a platform for greyhounds to compete for prestige and acclaim on Scottish soil.

The American Classics:

1. The Greyhound Night of Stars: Hosted at the Phoenix Greyhound Park in Arizona, the Greyhound Night of Stars is a celebrated American event that brings together top greyhounds for a night of electrifying competition. With various categories and substantial prize money, this event has become a highlight on the American racing calendar, drawing spectators and participants alike.

2. The Daytona 550: As one of the premier events in the United States, the Daytona 550 is held at the iconic Daytona Beach Kennel Club. The 550-yard race is a showcase of speed and endurance, and winning this event is a testament to a greyhound's exceptional abilities. The Daytona 550 continues to capture the imagination of racing enthusiasts across the nation.

International Showcases:

1. Melbourne Cup for Greyhounds: Inspired by the famed horse race, the Melbourne Cup for Greyhounds is a prestigious Australian event held at Sandown Park. Greyhounds from across Australia and beyond converge on the track to vie for this coveted title. The Melbourne Cup for Greyhounds has become synonymous with the excitement and allure of Australian greyhound racing.

2. The Irish Laurels: A key fixture in the Irish racing calendar, the Irish Laurels is a highlight at Cork's Curraheen Park. This classic event, established in 1949, has witnessed legendary performances and fierce competition. The Irish

Laurels continues to attract top-tier talent, showcasing the best of Irish greyhound racing.

Distinctive Prizes and Trophies:

1. The Easter Cup: Held annually at Shelbourne Park in Ireland, the Easter Cup is not only a classic race but also a prestigious prize in its own right. The winner not only secures a place in racing history but also takes home the coveted Easter Cup trophy, symbolizing excellence and achievement in the sport.

2. The Greyhound Grand National: The Greyhound Grand National, hosted at Sittingbourne Stadium in England, is a unique event that combines both flat and hurdle racing. Greyhounds must display versatility and skill as they navigate the different challenges posed by this distinctive competition. The Grand National trophy represents the pinnacle of success in this demanding event.

The Pursuit of Prestige:

1. Brisbane Cup: In the Southern Hemisphere, the Brisbane Cup holds a distinguished status in Australian greyhound racing. Conducted at Albion Park, this classic race is steeped in history and tradition. The Brisbane Cup trophy symbolizes the pursuit of excellence and is a cherished prize in the world of Australian greyhound racing.

2. The Puppy Derby: As a showcase for emerging talent, the Puppy Derby is a classic race that highlights the potential stars of the future. Held at various tracks around the world, including Wimbledon Stadium in England, the Puppy Derby provides a platform for young greyhounds to make their mark and aspire to greatness in the sport.

The Enigma of the Eclipse Awards:

1. Eclipse Awards for Greyhounds: Inspired by the prestigious Thoroughbred racing awards, the Eclipse Awards for Greyhounds recognize outstanding achievements in the sport. This accolade, presented annually in the United States, encompasses various categories, including Greyhound of the Year and other noteworthy accomplishments. Winning an Eclipse Award is a testament to a greyhound's exceptional talent and contributions to the sport.

2. Golden Jacket: The Golden Jacket, an esteemed prize in the world of greyhound racing, is contested at Crayford Stadium in England. The winner not only receives the title of Golden Jacket champion but also claims the coveted trophy. This classic event attracts top contenders, and the Golden Jacket remains a sought-after accolade in the racing community.

The Essence of Championship Races:

1. Achieving Triple Crown Glory: In both the United States and Ireland, achieving the Greyhound Triple Crown—victory in three prestigious races within a specific timeframe—is a rare and coveted accomplishment. The Triple Crown comprises the English Greyhound Derby, the Irish Greyhound Derby, and the English Greyhound St. Leger. Greyhounds that attain Triple Crown glory etch their names in the echelons of racing greatness.

2. The St. Leger: The English Greyhound St. Leger, named after the classic horse race, is a defining event in the world of greyhound racing. Run at Wimbledon Stadium until its closure, and later at Perry Barr Stadium, the St. Leger has a

storied history dating back to 1928. Winning the St. Leger is a mark of distinction, and the trophy represents the pinnacle of success in this classic competition.

Conclusion - Icons Carved in History:

As we traverse the landscape of classic races and prizes in greyhound racing, it becomes evident that these events are more than competitions—they are the crucibles where legends are born, and the extraordinary is made ordinary. The trophies, awards, and accolades associated with these races serve as symbols of excellence, marking the indelible contributions of greyhounds, trainers, and the entire racing community to the rich tapestry of the sport. In the ensuing chapters, we will further explore the Hall of Fame greyhounds who have left an indelible mark on the sport and delve into the profiles of top racers from different eras.

Notable Racetracks that Host Premier Events

In the pulsating world of greyhound racing, the choice of racetrack is paramount. These venues are not merely arenas for competition; they are the theaters where the drama of speed, skill, and strategy unfolds. From historic tracks with a legacy spanning decades to modern facilities designed for the contemporary racing experience, the following section explores notable racetracks around the world that have earned their place as hosts of premier greyhound racing events.

1. Towcester Racecourse, England:

- Overview: Nestled in the heart of England, Towcester Racecourse boasts a rich history as one of the premier venues for greyhound racing. Originally opened in 1928, the track has witnessed the triumphs of legendary greyhounds in the English Greyhound Derby, an iconic event that has elevated Towcester to international acclaim.

- The English Greyhound Derby: Towcester Racecourse has been the traditional home of the English Greyhound Derby, an event that stands as a pinnacle in the sport. The expansive track, with its challenging turns and straightaways, provides the perfect stage for greyhounds to showcase their speed and agility. The English Greyhound Derby's association with Towcester is synonymous with the race's storied legacy.

2. Shelbourne Park, Dublin, Ireland:

- Overview: Situated in the vibrant city of Dublin, Shelbourne Park has been a cornerstone of Irish greyhound racing since its inauguration in 1927. The track combines tradition with modern amenities, offering a dynamic setting for both enthusiasts and competitors. Shelbourne Park is not only a venue for top-tier races but also a cultural hub for greyhound racing in Ireland.

- The Irish Greyhound Derby: Shelbourne Park takes center stage as the host of the Irish Greyhound Derby, an event that captivates the nation. The track's strategic layout and passionate crowd create an electric atmosphere for this premier race. Greyhounds that triumph at Shelbourne Park etch their names into the annals of Irish racing history.

3. Sandown Park, Melbourne, Australia:

- Overview: In the Southern Hemisphere, Sandown Park in Melbourne, Australia, stands as an iconic venue for greyhound racing. Established in 1935, Sandown Park has evolved into a state-of-the-art facility that marries a rich racing heritage with contemporary amenities. The track's distinctive triangular shape adds a unique dimension to the racing experience.

- Melbourne Cup for Greyhounds: Sandown Park hosts the prestigious Melbourne Cup for Greyhounds, an event that draws competitors from across Australia. The track's layout, with its sweeping turns and long straights, poses a thrilling challenge for greyhounds. The Melbourne Cup for Greyhounds at Sandown Park is a showcase of speed, skill, and determination.

4. Daytona Beach Kennel Club, United States:

- Overview: As a symbol of American racing excitement, the Daytona Beach Kennel Club in Florida has been a hub for greyhound enthusiasts since its establishment in 1948. The track's proximity to the iconic Daytona International Speedway adds a layer of excitement, creating a unique racing destination.

- The Daytona 550: The Daytona 550, held at the Daytona Beach Kennel Club, is a showcase of speed and skill over the 550-yard distance. The track's design, coupled with its association with the legendary Daytona Beach, infuses the event with a sense of spectacle. The Daytona 550 is a testament to the enduring appeal of greyhound racing in the United States.

5. Crayford Stadium, England:

- Overview: Crayford Stadium, located in the county of Kent, England, has been a fixture in the greyhound racing landscape since its opening in 1927. The track's consistent commitment to excellence has made it a favorite among racing enthusiasts, and its strategic design enhances the competitiveness of races.

- The Golden Jacket: Crayford Stadium hosts the esteemed Golden Jacket, a classic race that tests greyhounds over varying distances. The track's reputation for providing a fair yet challenging course makes the Golden Jacket a sought-after prize. Victory at Crayford Stadium signifies a greyhound's prowess and adaptability.

6. Phoenix Greyhound Park, United States:

- Overview: Phoenix Greyhound Park in Arizona, USA, has been a dynamic force in American greyhound racing since its opening in 1954. The track's strategic location and modern facilities contribute to its status as a premier racing destination in the southwestern United States.

- The Greyhound Night of Stars: Phoenix Greyhound Park hosts the Greyhound Night of Stars, an event that showcases top-tier talent from around the country. The Night of Stars, with its diverse categories and substantial prize money, elevates the profile of greyhound racing in the United States. The track's commitment to excellence is reflected in the caliber of competition it attracts.

7. Perry Barr Stadium, Birmingham, England:

- Overview: Perry Barr Stadium in Birmingham, England, has been a prominent fixture in the British greyhound racing scene since its establishment in 1929. The track's accessibility and modern amenities make it a popular choice for both racing participants and spectators.

- The English Greyhound St. Leger: Perry Barr Stadium is the venue for the English Greyhound St. Leger, a classic race that dates back to 1928. The St. Leger, with its blend of flat and hurdle racing, tests the versatility of greyhounds. Perry Barr Stadium's role in hosting this distinctive event underscores its significance in the British racing calendar.

8. Curraheen Park, Cork, Ireland:

- Overview: Curraheen Park, located in Cork, Ireland, is synonymous with the thrill of Irish greyhound racing. Since its opening in 1947, the track has been a beloved destination for enthusiasts and a stage for top-class competition. Curraheen Park's strategic layout contributes to the excitement of the races held on its hallowed grounds.

- The Irish Laurels: Curraheen Park is the proud host of the Irish Laurels, an event that has become a cornerstone of Irish racing tradition. The Laurels, with its esteemed history and challenging course, attracts the best greyhounds from Ireland and beyond. Curraheen Park's role in shaping the narrative of Irish greyhound racing is enshrined in the prestige of the Laurels.

9. Albion Park, Brisbane, Australia:

- Overview: Albion Park in Brisbane, Australia, is a testament to the global appeal of greyhound racing. Established in 1922, the track has undergone transformations to emerge as a modern racing facility. Albion Park's strategic design and commitment to high standards make it a preferred venue for top-tier competitions.

- Brisbane Cup: The Brisbane Cup, hosted at Albion Park, is a highlight in the Australian racing calendar. The Cup, with its prestigious history and generous prize purse, attracts elite greyhounds from across the country. Albion Park's role as the host of the Brisbane Cup underscores its significance in shaping the narrative of Australian greyhound racing.

10. Wimbledon Stadium, London, England:

- Overview: Wimbledon Stadium, in the heart of London, England, was a historic bastion of greyhound racing until its closure in 2017. The track's rich legacy and central location made it a cultural landmark for racing enthusiasts. While Wimbledon Stadium is no longer operational, its influence on the sport remains indelible.

- The English Greyhound St. Leger and Puppy Derby: Wimbledon Stadium played a crucial role in hosting the English Greyhound St. Leger and the Puppy Derby, events that defined the British racing calendar. The St. Leger's blend of flat and hurdle racing and the Puppy Derby's focus on emerging talent made Wimbledon Stadium a hub for diverse racing experiences.

Conclusion - Tracks of Endurance and Legacy:

Notable racetracks serve as more than just venues for competition; they are theaters where the stories of greyhound racing unfold. The iconic tracks highlighted in this chapter have etched their names into the sport's history, hosting premier events that capture the imagination of racing enthusiasts worldwide. Each track brings a unique flavor to the racing experience, whether it be the tradition-laden history of Towcester or the modern allure of Sandown Park. As we delve deeper into the world of greyhound racing, the tracks we explore will continue to shape the narrative of this thrilling and enduring sport.

Hall of Fame Greyhounds Through History

In the illustrious tapestry of greyhound racing, certain athletes transcend the boundaries of their time, leaving an indelible mark on the sport. These are the Hall of Fame greyhounds—extraordinary competitors whose prowess, resilience, and sheer speed have etched their names into the annals of racing history. This chapter pays homage to these iconic canines, exploring their achievements, contributions, and the enduring legacy they've left on the world of greyhound racing.

1. Mick the Miller (1926–1939):

- Background: Mick the Miller, a Greyhound of the Century awardee, stands as a legendary figure in the early days of greyhound racing. Born in 1926 in Ireland, Mick captured the public's imagination with his exceptional speed and record-breaking performances.

- Achievements: Mick's racing career included victories in prestigious events like the English Greyhound Derby in 1929 and 1930. His remarkable ability to cover ground with unparalleled speed made him a crowd favorite and an enduring symbol of racing excellence.

- Legacy: Mick the Miller's legacy extends beyond the track. His impact on the sport elevated greyhound racing to new heights, and his name remains synonymous with the golden age of early 20th-century racing.

2. Ballyregan Bob (1977–1984):

- Background: Ballyregan Bob, born in 1977, was a greyhound of exceptional talent and endurance. Hailing from

Ireland, Bob became a dominant force in British greyhound racing during the late 1970s and early 1980s.

- Achievements: Bob's list of achievements is impressive, including winning the English Greyhound Derby in 1980 and securing numerous track records. His relentless pursuit of victory and remarkable consistency set him apart as one of the greatest racers of his era.

- Legacy: Ballyregan Bob's legacy is marked by his influence on breeding and racing standards. His bloodline continues to impact the greyhound racing landscape, and his name is revered among enthusiasts and breeders alike.

3. Westmead Hawk (1998–2006):

- Background: Westmead Hawk, born in 1998, emerged as a dominant force in greyhound racing during the late 1990s and early 2000s. Bred in Ireland, Hawk showcased a rare combination of speed, agility, and racing intelligence.

- Achievements: Hawk's list of accomplishments includes winning the English Greyhound Derby in 2001 and achieving a world record time for 480 meters. His electrifying performances on the track solidified his status as a modern-day racing legend.

- Legacy: Westmead Hawk's legacy extends to his influence on the perception of greyhounds as athletes. His achievements elevated the profile of greyhound racing, attracting new fans and cementing his place among the sport's all-time greats.

4. Rapid Ranger (1986–1995):

- Background: Rapid Ranger, born in 1986, was a greyhound renowned for his remarkable racing career in the

United States. Bred in Ireland and later exported to the U.S., Ranger left an indelible mark on American greyhound racing.

- Achievements: Ranger's achievements include winning the prestigious Hollywoodian Stakes and the American Derby. His ability to excel on both dirt and grass tracks showcased his versatility and racing prowess.

- Legacy: Rapid Ranger's legacy extends to his impact on international greyhound racing. His success in the United States contributed to the globalization of the sport, inspiring greyhound enthusiasts worldwide.

5. Greyhound of the Year (Various):

- Overview: The title of Greyhound of the Year is awarded to the canine athlete that exemplifies excellence in a given year. Various greyhounds have earned this accolade through exceptional performances, consistency, and sportsmanship.

- Achievements: Greyhounds of the Year often have diverse accomplishments, ranging from winning major races to setting track records. These athletes symbolize the pinnacle of racing achievement in their respective years.

- Legacy: The legacy of Greyhound of the Year recipients is intertwined with the evolving narrative of greyhound racing. Each winner contributes to the sport's rich history and inspires future generations of competitors.

6. Other Hall of Fame Inductees:

- Dyna Tron (1996–2003): Dyna Tron, an Australian greyhound, achieved success in the late 1990s, winning the Melbourne Cup and the Topgun.

- Patricia's Hope (1978–1983): Patricia's Hope, a female greyhound, made history by winning the English Greyhound Derby in 1980.

- Kingsfield Andy (1982–1990): Kingsfield Andy, an Irish greyhound, left a lasting legacy with victories in the Irish Greyhound Derby and the Grand National.

Conclusion - Legends on the Track:

The Hall of Fame greyhounds highlighted in this chapter are not merely athletes; they are icons who have shaped the narrative of greyhound racing. Their exceptional abilities, tenacity, and enduring legacy have elevated the sport to new heights. As we delve deeper into the world of greyhound racing, we will continue to explore the stories of these racing legends and the profound impact they have had on the sport we celebrate and cherish.

Profiles of Top Racers from Past Eras

In the annals of greyhound racing, the sport's rich history is woven with the tales of exceptional athletes whose prowess on the track captivated audiences and left an enduring legacy. This chapter delves into the profiles of some of the top racers from past eras, exploring their achievements, racing styles, and the impact they had on the landscape of greyhound racing.

1. Mick the Miller (1926–1939):

- Overview: Mick the Miller, a greyhound of legendary status, rose to prominence in the early 20th century. Born in 1926 in Ireland, Mick became a symbol of speed and endurance, capturing the hearts of racing enthusiasts worldwide.

- Racing Style: Mick the Miller was known for his explosive starts and the ability to maintain a relentless pace throughout races. His distinctive style, marked by powerful strides and strategic prowess, set the standard for greyhound racing in his era.

- Key Achievements: Mick's list of achievements includes back-to-back victories in the English Greyhound Derby in 1929 and 1930. His record-breaking performances and consistent success established him as one of the greatest racers of the early greyhound racing age.

2. Patricias Hope (1978–1983):

- Overview: Patricias Hope, a female greyhound, made history in the late 1970s and early 1980s. Born in 1978, she defied expectations and etched her name in the annals of the English Greyhound Derby.

- Racing Style: Patricias Hope was renowned for her agility and strategic acumen on the track. Despite facing male competitors in the English Greyhound Derby, she showcased remarkable speed and determination, earning the admiration of fans and competitors alike.

- Key Achievements: Patricias Hope's crowning achievement came in 1980 when she became the first and, to date, the only female greyhound to win the English Greyhound Derby. Her triumph shattered gender norms and solidified her place in greyhound racing history.

3. Rapid Ranger (1986–1995):

- Overview: Rapid Ranger, born in 1986, left an indelible mark on American greyhound racing during the late 1980s and early 1990s. Bred in Ireland, Ranger showcased versatility and excellence on both dirt and grass tracks.

- Racing Style: Rapid Ranger's racing style was characterized by his adaptability to different track conditions. Whether it was a dirt or grass track, he exhibited a potent combination of speed, agility, and strategic intelligence.

- Key Achievements: Ranger's impressive list of achievements includes victories in the prestigious Hollywoodian Stakes and the American Derby. His success contributed to the globalization of greyhound racing, inspiring enthusiasts around the world.

4. Westmead Hawk (1998–2006):

- Overview: Westmead Hawk, born in 1998, emerged as a dominant force in greyhound racing during the late 1990s and early 2000s. Hailing from Ireland, Hawk's exceptional abilities made him a modern-day racing legend.

- Racing Style: Westmead Hawk's racing style was characterized by explosive starts and a strong finishing kick. His strategic acumen allowed him to navigate races with precision, making him a formidable competitor.

- Key Achievements: Hawk's list of achievements includes winning the English Greyhound Derby in 2001 and achieving a world record time for 480 meters. His electrifying performances on the track solidified his status as one of the greatest greyhounds of his era.

5. Ballyregan Bob (1977–1984):

- Overview: Ballyregan Bob, born in 1977, was a greyhound of extraordinary talent and endurance. Originating from Ireland, Bob's dominance in British greyhound racing during the late 1970s and early 1980s is etched in racing history.

- Racing Style: Ballyregan Bob's racing style was marked by relentless pursuit and consistent performances. His ability to maintain high speeds over varying distances made him a standout competitor.

- Key Achievements: Bob's list of achievements includes winning the English Greyhound Derby in 1980 and setting numerous track records. His legacy extends to his impact on breeding standards, with his bloodline influencing the sport for years to come.

6. Other Racing Icons:

- Dyna Tron (1996–2003): Dyna Tron, an Australian greyhound, achieved success in the late 1990s, winning the Melbourne Cup and the Topgun.

- Kingsfield Andy (1982–1990): Kingsfield Andy, an Irish greyhound, left a lasting legacy with victories in the Irish Greyhound Derby and the Grand National.

- Greyhound of the Year Recipients (Various): Various greyhounds have earned the title of Greyhound of the Year, symbolizing excellence in their respective years and contributing to the sport's vibrant history.

Conclusion - Racing Legends Across Eras:

The profiles of these top racers from past eras offer a glimpse into the diverse and rich history of greyhound racing. Each of these athletes, with their unique styles and remarkable achievements, has left an indelible mark on the sport. As we celebrate their legacies, we also honor the broader narrative of greyhound racing, shaped by the speed, skill, and spirit of these exceptional competitors.

Current Rising Stars and Fan Favorites

As the world of greyhound racing evolves, a new generation of canine athletes emerges to carry the torch of excitement, skill, and competition. This chapter introduces the current rising stars and fan favorites, exploring their achievements, racing styles, and the enthusiastic following they've garnered from audiences around the globe.

1. Rising Stars:

- Overview: The realm of greyhound racing is continually rejuvenated by the emergence of rising stars— athletes that captivate audiences with their raw talent and untapped potential. These young greyhounds bring a fresh energy to the sport, enticing fans with the promise of thrilling races and record-breaking performances.

- Noteworthy Rising Stars:

- Swift Thunder: A young greyhound known for lightning-fast starts and an impressive sprinting ability.

- Silver Streak: Gaining attention for consistent podium finishes and a remarkable aptitude for navigating turns.

- Blaze of Glory: A rising star with a fiery racing style, showing a competitive edge in both short and long-distance races.

2. Fan Favorites:

- Overview: Beyond sheer racing prowess, certain greyhounds capture the hearts of fans through their charisma, unique personalities, and memorable racing moments. These fan favorites become more than athletes; they become icons of the sport, creating lasting connections with audiences worldwide.

- Beloved Fan Favorites:

- Spirit of the Track: Known for a resilient racing spirit and a never-give-up attitude, earning the admiration of fans.

- Midnight Mirage: A striking black-coated greyhound with a captivating presence, drawing fans to the track with anticipation.

- Heart's Symphony: A fan favorite celebrated for a harmonious blend of speed, agility, and a joyful demeanor both on and off the track.

3. Notable Achievements:

- Swift Thunder's Streak of Victories: Swift Thunder has been on an impressive winning streak, claiming victory in multiple prestigious races and showcasing a remarkable consistency that has fans eagerly anticipating each race.

- Silver Streak's Record-Breaking Turns: Silver Streak has gained acclaim for mastering the art of navigating turns with unparalleled agility. Setting records for turn speed, this fan favorite has added a dynamic element to greyhound racing.

- Blaze of Glory's Versatility: Blaze of Glory has emerged as a versatile racer, excelling in both short sprints and longer-distance races. This adaptability has endeared the greyhound to a diverse fan base, appreciating the thrill of varied racing challenges.

4. Racing Styles:

- Swift Thunder's Lightning Starts: Swift Thunder's racing style is characterized by explosive starts, often leaving competitors trailing in the opening moments of a race. This swift acceleration has become a signature move, earning the greyhound a reputation for lightning-fast performances.

- Silver Streak's Graceful Turns: Silver Streak's racing style stands out in the artful execution of turns. Navigating bends with grace and precision, the greyhound has redefined the approach to cornering, setting a new standard for agility on the track.

- Blaze of Glory's Fearless Pursuit: Blaze of Glory's racing style is marked by a fearless pursuit of victory. Whether chasing down rivals or maintaining a steady lead, this greyhound's determination and competitive spirit have become defining features of its racing persona.

5. International Appeal:

- Swift Thunder's Global Following: Swift Thunder's electrifying performances have garnered a global following, with fans tuning in from various continents to witness the greyhound's speed and agility. This international appeal has added a new dimension to the sport's global reach.

- Silver Streak's Charismatic Presence: Silver Streak's charismatic presence transcends borders, attracting fans from diverse cultures who appreciate the greyhound's unique racing style. The greyhound's popularity extends to international racing events, where spectators eagerly await its appearances.

- Blaze of Glory's Online Fan Communities: Blaze of Glory has inspired the creation of online fan communities, bringing together enthusiasts to share highlights, discuss races, and celebrate the greyhound's achievements. The sense of community adds a digital dimension to the fan base, connecting followers from around the world.

6. Behind-the-Scenes Stories:

- Swift Thunder's Training Regimen: Delving into Swift Thunder's training regimen reveals the meticulous preparation that goes into optimizing the greyhound's performance. From specialized workouts to tailored nutrition plans, the behind-the-scenes story provides insight into the dedication of trainers and handlers.

- Silver Streak's Bond with Handlers: Silver Streak's close bond with handlers is a heartwarming aspect of the behind-the-scenes narrative. The trust and connection between the greyhound and its human companions contribute to the overall racing experience and deepen the emotional connection with fans.

- Blaze of Glory's Off-Track Personality: Exploring Blaze of Glory's off-track personality sheds light on the playful and affectionate side of the greyhound. Beyond the intensity of races, fans get a glimpse into the daily life and character of this fan favorite, fostering a deeper connection with the audience.

Conclusion - Embracing the Future:

As current rising stars and fan favorites continue to shape the landscape of greyhound racing, the sport enters a new era of excitement and anticipation. The stories of these greyhounds, with their unique racing styles and the devoted communities they inspire, contribute to the rich tapestry of greyhound racing's evolving narrative. As we celebrate their achievements, we also look ahead to the future, where new stars will emerge, and the spirit of competition will endure.

Chapter 5: Controversies and Animal Welfare
Injuries and Health Issues for Racing Greyhounds

While greyhound racing is a thrilling and deeply rooted sport, it has not been without controversy, particularly concerning the welfare of the canine athletes involved. This chapter delves into the complex issues surrounding injuries and health concerns for racing greyhounds, shedding light on the challenges faced by these remarkable animals in the pursuit of speed and victory.

1. Physical Strain of Racing:

- Overview: The intense nature of greyhound racing places considerable physical strain on the athletes. From the explosive starts to the high-speed pursuits around the track, racing greyhounds experience immense stress on their bodies. Understanding the specific physical demands helps illuminate the potential for injuries and health issues.

- Impact on Musculoskeletal System: The musculoskeletal system, including bones, joints, and muscles, bears the brunt of the physical demands of racing. The rapid acceleration, sudden turns, and the sheer force of running at high speeds can lead to stress on joints and an increased risk of injuries, such as sprains and fractures.

2. Common Injuries in Greyhound Racing:

- Fractures: Fractures, particularly of the limbs, are among the most common injuries in greyhound racing. The sheer speed and agility required during races elevate the risk of bone fractures, necessitating immediate veterinary attention.

- Muscle Strains: The explosive bursts of acceleration and deceleration put strain on the muscles, increasing the likelihood of strains. Muscle injuries can affect the greyhound's performance and may require rehabilitation to ensure a full recovery.

- Ligament Injuries: Ligaments, crucial for joint stability, are susceptible to injury during the intense and dynamic movements of racing. Common ligament injuries include sprains or tears, impacting the greyhound's ability to race effectively.

- Foot and Paw Issues: The repeated pounding on the track surface can lead to foot and paw issues, including abrasions, lacerations, and the development of conditions like corns. Foot problems can affect a greyhound's gait and overall well-being.

3. Health Issues Related to Racing:

- Cardiovascular Stress: Greyhound racing demands a significant cardiovascular effort, placing stress on the heart and circulatory system. While these athletes are well-conditioned, the persistent high-intensity exercise can contribute to cardiovascular issues over time.

- Respiratory Strain: The rapid breathing required during races, combined with the inhalation of dust and particles from the track, can lead to respiratory strain. Conditions like exercise-induced pulmonary hemorrhage may occur, affecting the greyhound's respiratory health.

- Dehydration and Heat Stress: Racing, often conducted in various weather conditions, can expose greyhounds to the risk of dehydration and heat stress. Maintaining hydration is crucial, and extreme temperatures can pose challenges to the greyhound's thermoregulatory mechanisms.

4. Veterinary Care and Injury Prevention:

- Pre-Race Health Assessments: Rigorous pre-race health assessments are essential to identify any underlying issues that might compromise a greyhound's well-being during a race. Regular veterinary check-ups, including musculoskeletal evaluations, help ensure the athletes are fit for competition.

- Injury Rehabilitation Programs: When injuries occur, prompt and effective rehabilitation programs are crucial for the greyhound's recovery. These programs may include rest, physiotherapy, and controlled exercise to facilitate healing and prevent long-term consequences.

- Improved Track Surfaces: Investing in improved track surfaces can contribute to injury prevention. Surfaces that provide adequate traction, shock absorption, and are well-maintained reduce the impact on a greyhound's musculoskeletal system, mitigating the risk of injuries.

5. Ethical Considerations:

- Balancing Competition and Welfare: Striking a balance between the competitive nature of greyhound racing and the welfare of the athletes is a complex ethical consideration. Advocates for greyhound welfare emphasize the need for stringent regulations and ethical practices to protect these animals.

- Industry Responsibility: The greyhound racing industry bears a responsibility to prioritize the health and well-being of its participants. Implementing and enforcing comprehensive welfare standards, alongside transparent reporting of injuries, is essential to address ethical concerns.

6. Advances in Greyhound Health Research:

- Genetic Screening: Genetic screening is advancing as a tool to identify potential health issues in greyhounds. Understanding genetic predispositions can aid in selective breeding practices and minimize the risk of hereditary conditions.

- Nutritional Science: Research in nutritional science is focusing on optimizing diets to support the unique nutritional needs of racing greyhounds. Proper nutrition is a key factor in maintaining overall health and reducing the risk of certain conditions.

- Rehabilitation Techniques: Advances in rehabilitation techniques, including physical therapy and alternative therapies such as hydrotherapy, are enhancing the recovery process for injured greyhounds. These techniques contribute to improved overall health and longevity.

Conclusion - Striving for a Balanced Future:

Navigating the controversies surrounding injuries and health issues for racing greyhounds requires a holistic approach that considers both the competitive aspects of the sport and the ethical responsibility to safeguard the well-being of these remarkable athletes. As the industry evolves, ongoing efforts in research, veterinary care, and ethical standards will play a crucial role in striving for a future where greyhound racing can coexist with the highest standards of animal welfare.

Scientific Studies on Breed Welfare

The welfare of racing greyhounds is a topic of considerable debate and concern within the broader context of greyhound racing. This chapter delves into the scientific studies conducted to assess and understand the welfare implications for racing greyhounds. By examining research findings, we aim to provide an evidence-based perspective on the physical, behavioral, and overall well-being of these canine athletes.

1. Physical Health and Musculoskeletal Studies:

- Bones and Joint Health: Scientific studies have explored the impact of racing on the bones and joints of greyhounds. Radiographic imaging and biomechanical analyses have been employed to assess the structural integrity of the musculoskeletal system, shedding light on the prevalence of fractures, sprains, and other related injuries.

- Gait Analysis: Gait analysis studies aim to understand the biomechanics of a greyhound's stride during racing. High-speed cameras and motion capture technology have been utilized to examine the gait patterns, joint angles, and ground reaction forces. These analyses provide valuable insights into the stresses placed on the musculoskeletal system.

- Effect of Track Surfaces: Research has investigated the influence of different track surfaces on greyhound health. Comparative studies assess the impact of surfaces on factors such as traction, shock absorption, and the occurrence of injuries. Findings contribute to recommendations for optimizing track conditions to reduce the risk of musculoskeletal issues.

2. Cardiovascular and Respiratory Health Studies:

- Heart Function during Racing: Cardiovascular studies have focused on the heart function of racing greyhounds during exercise. Echocardiography and heart rate monitoring provide data on cardiac performance, helping to understand the cardiovascular demands placed on these athletes. Findings contribute to discussions on the cardiovascular health of racing greyhounds.

- Respiratory Performance: Scientific investigations assess the respiratory health of greyhounds during races. Studies use techniques such as endoscopy and respiratory rate monitoring to evaluate the impact of high-intensity exercise on the respiratory system. This research is crucial in identifying potential issues and implementing measures to support respiratory well-being.

3. Behavioral Welfare Studies:

- Stress and Anxiety: Behavioral studies aim to assess stress and anxiety levels in racing greyhounds. Observational methods, cortisol level measurements, and behavioral questionnaires contribute to understanding how the racing environment, including pre-race activities and post-race experiences, may impact the psychological well-being of the greyhounds.

- Social Dynamics in Kennels: Research explores the social dynamics within racing kennels to understand the impact of kennel life on greyhound welfare. Observations of interactions between greyhounds, as well as the influence of kennel size and design, contribute to recommendations for creating environments that support positive social experiences.

- Retirement Transition: Studies investigate the transition of greyhounds from racing to retirement. Behavioral assessments and long-term follow-ups provide insights into the adaptation process, potential stressors during retirement, and strategies to facilitate a smooth transition to post-racing life.

4. Nutritional and Reproductive Health Studies:

- Nutritional Requirements: Nutritional studies focus on identifying the specific dietary needs of racing greyhounds. Assessments of nutrient requirements, including protein, fats, and vitamins, contribute to optimizing diets that support overall health, performance, and recovery.

- Reproductive Impacts: Research explores the reproductive health of racing greyhounds, considering factors such as breeding practices and the impact of racing on reproductive systems. Findings contribute to discussions on responsible breeding practices and the welfare considerations for breeding greyhounds.

5. Longitudinal Studies and Lifespan Analysis:

- Longitudinal Health Monitoring: Longitudinal studies track the health and well-being of racing greyhounds over extended periods. These comprehensive analyses provide valuable data on the cumulative effects of racing, aging, and potential post-retirement health issues.

- Lifespan Analysis: Research on the lifespan of racing greyhounds contributes to understanding the longevity of these athletes. Factors such as retirement age, post-racing care, and specific health conditions affecting lifespan are explored to inform practices that promote the well-being of greyhounds throughout their lives.

6. Implications for Industry Practices:

- Welfare-Driven Regulations: The findings from scientific studies have implications for industry regulations and practices. Welfare-driven regulations may be informed by evidence-based recommendations, covering aspects such as track conditions, training methods, and retirement protocols.

- Education and Best Practices: Scientific research contributes to educational initiatives for industry stakeholders, including owners, trainers, and track officials. Best practices informed by research findings can be disseminated to enhance the overall welfare of racing greyhounds.

Conclusion - Navigating the Welfare Landscape:

Scientific studies on breed welfare are invaluable tools in navigating the complex landscape of greyhound racing controversies. As research continues to provide nuanced insights into the physical and behavioral aspects of racing greyhounds, the industry is poised to make informed decisions that prioritize the welfare of these remarkable canine athletes. The collaborative efforts of researchers, industry professionals, and advocates contribute to a future where greyhound racing coexists with the highest standards of animal welfare.

Doping Scandals and Prevention Efforts

Greyhound racing, like many competitive sports, has not been immune to the controversies surrounding the use of performance-enhancing substances. This chapter delves into the world of doping scandals within the greyhound racing industry and the ongoing efforts to prevent the illicit use of substances that compromise the integrity of the sport and the welfare of the canine athletes.

1. Historical Context of Doping in Greyhound Racing:

- Early Instances: Doping scandals in greyhound racing date back to the early years of the sport. The use of stimulants, anabolic steroids, and other performance-enhancing substances has been documented, raising ethical concerns and prompting regulatory responses.

- Evolution of Doping Methods: The methods employed for doping greyhounds have evolved over time, paralleling advancements in sports science and pharmacology. From traditional stimulants to more sophisticated substances, the landscape of doping has become increasingly complex.

2. Impact on Greyhound Welfare:

- Health Consequences: Doping can have severe health consequences for racing greyhounds. The administration of certain substances, especially when done without proper veterinary oversight, may lead to cardiovascular issues, musculoskeletal problems, and long-term health complications.

- Performance Pressures: The use of performance-enhancing drugs creates an environment of intense competition, where trainers and owners may feel pressured to achieve consistent victories. This can contribute to a culture of doping as individuals seek an edge in the pursuit of success on the racetrack.

3. High-Profile Doping Scandals:

- Notable Cases: Examining high-profile doping scandals within greyhound racing sheds light on the magnitude of the issue. Instances of prominent trainers and owners facing sanctions due to doping violations have garnered public attention and raised questions about the efficacy of current preventive measures.

- Impact on Public Perception: Doping scandals have a significant impact on the public perception of greyhound racing. The loss of public trust, coupled with concerns about the welfare of the animals, has prompted calls for increased transparency, accountability, and stricter regulation.

4. Regulatory Responses and Anti-Doping Measures:

- Drug Testing Protocols: Regulatory bodies within the greyhound racing industry have implemented comprehensive drug testing protocols to detect banned substances. Urine and blood samples are routinely collected from racing greyhounds, and laboratories conduct analyses to identify the presence of prohibited drugs.

- Establishment of Anti-Doping Agencies: The establishment of anti-doping agencies dedicated to greyhound racing reflects a commitment to eradicating doping practices. These agencies work in collaboration with regulatory bodies to enforce anti-doping measures, conduct investigations, and ensure a level playing field for all participants.

- Stricter Penalties and Sanctions: Efforts to deter doping include the imposition of stricter penalties and sanctions for offenders. Increasing fines, suspensions, and disqualifications aim to create a deterrent effect and signal a commitment to maintaining the integrity of the sport.

5. Education and Awareness Initiatives:

- Trainer and Owner Education: Education initiatives target trainers and owners, providing information on the dangers of doping and the ethical considerations associated with compromising the welfare of racing greyhounds. Training programs emphasize the importance of fair competition and responsible care.

- Public Awareness Campaigns: Public awareness campaigns play a crucial role in fostering a culture of transparency and accountability. By informing the public about the risks and consequences of doping, these campaigns seek to generate support for stringent anti-doping measures.

6. Technological Advances in Detection:

- Advancements in Testing Technology: Technological innovations have played a pivotal role in enhancing the accuracy and efficiency of drug testing. Advances in testing technology, including mass spectrometry and other analytical methods, contribute to the detection of a wider range of substances.

- Biological Passport Systems: The introduction of biological passport systems in greyhound racing enables the monitoring of biological markers over time. This approach provides a comprehensive profile of each racing greyhound, facilitating the early detection of irregularities that may indicate doping.

7. Global Collaboration:

- International Cooperation: Given the global nature of greyhound racing, international cooperation is essential in combating doping. Collaborative efforts among racing jurisdictions, regulatory bodies, and anti-doping agencies contribute to a unified approach in addressing doping challenges.

- Information Sharing: The sharing of information and intelligence regarding doping practices is a key aspect of global collaboration. Rapid communication and coordinated responses enhance the ability of the industry to identify and address emerging threats to the integrity of greyhound racing.

8. Challenges and Future Directions:

- Evolution of Doping Methods: The constant evolution of doping methods poses an ongoing challenge for regulators and anti-doping agencies. Staying ahead of emerging substances and techniques requires continuous adaptation and innovation in testing protocols.

- Cultural Shift: Achieving a cultural shift within the industry, where doping is universally condemned, is a long-term goal. Education, strict enforcement, and a commitment to the welfare of racing greyhounds contribute to fostering a culture that prioritizes fair competition and ethical practices.

Conclusion - Safeguarding the Integrity and Welfare:

Doping scandals in greyhound racing represent a complex challenge that requires vigilance, collaboration, and a commitment to the welfare of the animals. The industry's response, marked by stringent anti-doping measures, technological advancements, and global cooperation, reflects a dedication to safeguarding the integrity of greyhound racing and ensuring the well-being of its extraordinary athletes.

Ethics of Breeding Practices and Culling

The ethical considerations surrounding the breeding practices and culling within the greyhound racing industry are at the forefront of discussions on the welfare of these remarkable canine athletes. This chapter explores the complex landscape of breeding, addressing the challenges and controversies associated with selective breeding, overpopulation concerns, and the difficult decisions surrounding culling.

1. Selective Breeding in Greyhound Racing:

- Objective of Selective Breeding: The primary objective of selective breeding in greyhound racing is to produce individuals with optimal racing traits, including speed, endurance, and agility. Breeders aim to enhance desirable characteristics while minimizing genetic factors that may compromise racing performance.

- Influence of Genetics on Racing Ability: Understanding the genetic basis of racing traits is essential for successful selective breeding. Research into the heritability of speed, stamina, and other performance-related attributes informs breeding decisions and contributes to the development of racing bloodlines.

2. Desirable Qualities in Racing Greyhounds:

- Physical Attributes: Selective breeding emphasizes physical attributes such as body structure, muscle composition, and skeletal conformation. The goal is to produce greyhounds with optimal biomechanics, facilitating efficient and injury-resistant racing.

- Temperament and Behavioral Traits: Beyond physical characteristics, temperament and behavioral traits are integral to racing success. Selective breeding aims to cultivate traits such as focus, drive, and adaptability, ensuring that racing greyhounds exhibit the necessary behaviors for competition.

- Health Considerations: Ethical breeding practices prioritize the overall health and well-being of racing greyhounds. Genetic screenings and health assessments contribute to breeding decisions, aiming to reduce the incidence of hereditary conditions and promote the longevity of the athletes.

3. Overpopulation Concerns and Responsible Breeding:

- Overbreeding and Excess Greyhounds: The rapid breeding of greyhounds to meet racing demands has led to concerns of overpopulation. The surplus of greyhounds, particularly those deemed unfit for racing, raises ethical dilemmas regarding the responsibility of breeders to ensure the well-being of every individual produced.

- Responsible Breeding Practices: Ethical breeders advocate for responsible practices that prioritize the quality of breeding over quantity. This includes careful consideration of the demand for racing greyhounds, ensuring that each greyhound bred is given the opportunity for a purposeful life, whether in racing or as a companion animal.

- Adoption Programs and Retraining Initiatives: To address overpopulation concerns, responsible breeders actively support adoption programs and retraining initiatives. These efforts contribute to finding suitable homes and alternative careers for greyhounds that may not excel in racing or have completed their racing careers.

4. Culling Practices in Greyhound Racing:

- Definition and Rationale: Culling, the selective euthanasia or disposal of greyhounds, is a controversial aspect of the industry. The rationale behind culling is often rooted in the pursuit of maintaining a competitive and successful racing program, with the goal of ensuring that only the most promising athletes continue in the sport.

- Ethical Concerns: Culling raises significant ethical concerns, as decisions about the fate of individual greyhounds are often influenced by performance, injuries, or economic considerations. Critics argue that culling may compromise the moral responsibility to prioritize the welfare of each greyhound, irrespective of their racing potential.

5. Alternatives to Culling:

- Retirement and Adoption Programs: An alternative to culling involves robust retirement and adoption programs. Ethical racing entities prioritize the humane retirement of greyhounds, facilitating their transition to post-racing life as companion animals. Adoption programs play a crucial role in finding loving homes for retired athletes.

- Reevaluation of Racing Careers: Some argue for a reevaluation of racing careers, promoting a more flexible approach that considers the individual needs and capabilities of greyhounds. This may involve assessing each greyhound's suitability for different racing distances, adapting training regimens, or exploring alternative roles.

6. Industry Reforms and Welfare Standards:

- Regulatory Oversight: The implementation of regulatory oversight and welfare standards is critical in addressing ethical concerns within the industry. Regulatory bodies play a pivotal role in establishing guidelines for breeding practices, culling decisions, and overall welfare standards for racing greyhounds.

- Transparency and Accountability: Industry reforms often center on improving transparency and accountability. Establishing clear reporting mechanisms, ensuring public access to information, and holding stakeholders accountable for ethical breaches contribute to a culture of responsible and humane practices.

7. Public Perception and Advocacy:

- Impact of Public Awareness: Public awareness and advocacy efforts play a crucial role in influencing industry practices. Increased awareness of ethical considerations, including breeding practices and culling, prompts public scrutiny and encourages the industry to align with evolving societal values.

- Collaboration with Animal Welfare Organizations: Collaboration with animal welfare organizations fosters a collective approach to addressing ethical challenges. By working together, industry stakeholders and advocacy groups can develop and implement initiatives that prioritize the welfare of racing greyhounds.

Conclusion - Balancing Tradition and Ethics:

Navigating the ethical landscape of breeding practices and culling requires a delicate balance between the tradition of greyhound racing and evolving ethical standards. Industry stakeholders, breeders, regulators, and the public must collaborate to establish practices that prioritize the welfare of these extraordinary athletes, ensuring a future where greyhound racing aligns with the highest ethical standards and societal expectations.

Retirement and Adoption of Former Racers

The retirement and adoption of former racing greyhounds represent a crucial aspect of the ethical considerations within the greyhound racing industry. This chapter delves into the challenges and opportunities associated with the transition of these canine athletes from the racetrack to their post-racing lives, exploring initiatives, best practices, and the evolving landscape of retirement and adoption programs.

1. The Transition from Racing to Retirement:

- Importance of Thoughtful Transitions: The transition from racing to retirement is a critical phase in a greyhound's life. Ethical considerations emphasize the need for thoughtful and humane transitions, recognizing the individual needs and preferences of each greyhound as they exit the competitive racing environment.

- Physical and Behavioral Adjustments: Greyhounds accustomed to the structured routine of racing may undergo physical and behavioral adjustments during retirement. Understanding these changes is essential for providing appropriate care, support, and retraining as they adapt to life outside the racetrack.

2. Initiatives Promoting Responsible Retirements:

- Industry-Supported Retirement Programs: Ethical racing entities actively support retirement programs designed to ensure the well-being of greyhounds post-racing. These programs often involve collaboration with adoption agencies, veterinary professionals, and trainers to facilitate a seamless transition.

- Financial Contributions to Retraining: Some racing entities contribute financially to retraining initiatives aimed at preparing greyhounds for non-racing roles. Financial support may cover expenses related to rehabilitation, retraining programs, and the provision of necessary medical care for retired athletes.

3. Adoption as Companion Animals:

- Adoption Processes and Criteria: Adoption processes for racing greyhounds typically involve thorough assessments of potential adopters to ensure a suitable match between the greyhound's needs and the adoptive home. Criteria may include living arrangements, commitment to veterinary care, and the provision of a safe and loving environment.

- Education and Support for Adopters: Ethical adoption programs prioritize the education and support of adopters. Informational resources, training materials, and ongoing assistance help adopters understand the unique characteristics and needs of retired racing greyhounds, fostering successful transitions to pet life.

4. Challenges in Retiring and Adopting Greyhounds:

- Volume of Retirements: The sheer volume of greyhounds retiring from racing poses logistical challenges for adoption programs. Managing retirements efficiently requires strategic planning, collaboration between racing entities and adoption agencies, and a commitment to finding suitable homes for all retired greyhounds.

- Public Perception and Stereotypes: Public perception and stereotypes about racing greyhounds may present challenges in the adoption process. Overcoming misconceptions and promoting the positive qualities of retired greyhounds are essential in facilitating successful adoptions and dispelling myths surrounding the breed.

5. Retraining Programs and Alternative Careers:

- Diverse Career Opportunities: Retraining programs explore the diverse career opportunities available to retired racing greyhounds. These may include participation in canine sports, therapy work, and service roles. By showcasing the versatility and adaptability of greyhounds, these programs contribute to changing perceptions about the breed.

- Collaboration with Canine Professionals: Collaboration with canine professionals, such as trainers experienced in non-racing activities, enhances the success of retraining programs. Leveraging the expertise of professionals ensures that retired greyhounds receive appropriate training and support as they explore alternative careers.

6. Advocacy for Greyhound Welfare in Retirement:

- Role of Animal Welfare Organizations: Animal welfare organizations play a pivotal role in advocating for the welfare of retired racing greyhounds. Through awareness campaigns, policy initiatives, and collaboration with industry stakeholders, these organizations contribute to shaping ethical retirement practices.

- Legislation and Regulation: Legislative efforts and regulatory measures may be introduced to ensure the welfare of retired greyhounds. This includes standards for post-racing care, the establishment of retirement funds, and regulations that promote responsible retirement and adoption practices.

7. Success Stories and Positive Outcomes:

- Highlighting Positive Transitions: Sharing success stories of retired greyhounds thriving in their post-racing lives contributes to changing perceptions and showcasing the positive outcomes of ethical retirement and adoption programs. These narratives emphasize the individuality and resilience of greyhounds in their transition to companion animals.

- Celebrating Adopter Experiences: Celebrating the experiences of adopters and their retired greyhounds fosters a sense of community and encourages others to consider adopting. Adopter testimonials, social media campaigns, and community events contribute to building a positive narrative around retired racing greyhounds.

8. Industry Collaboration for Ethical Transitions:

- Collaboration Between Racing Entities and Adoption Agencies: Ethical retirement and adoption require seamless collaboration between racing entities and adoption agencies. Shared resources, communication channels, and joint initiatives contribute to creating a comprehensive and ethical framework for the transition of greyhounds.

- Industry Standards and Best Practices: Establishing industry standards and best practices for retirement and adoption ensures a consistent and ethical approach across the greyhound racing community. By setting benchmarks for care, retraining, and adoption processes, the industry can prioritize the well-being of greyhounds beyond their racing careers.

Conclusion - Paving the Way for Dignified Retirements:

Retirement and adoption programs stand as crucial components of ethical greyhound racing practices. By prioritizing the dignified transition of these canine athletes to post-racing life, the industry can demonstrate its commitment to the welfare of racing greyhounds, fostering a culture of responsible care and ethical stewardship.

Chapter 6: Greyhound Breeding and Bloodlines
Desirable Qualities in Racing Greyhounds

The breeding of racing greyhounds is a meticulous and strategic process aimed at enhancing specific qualities that contribute to success on the racetrack. This chapter explores the desirable qualities sought after in racing greyhounds, emphasizing the physical, temperamental, and performance attributes that breeders carefully consider to produce elite athletes.

1. Speed and Acceleration:

- Foundation of Racing Success: Speed is a fundamental quality sought after in racing greyhounds. Breeding programs prioritize individuals with exceptional acceleration and top-end speed, as these attributes directly impact a greyhound's ability to outpace competitors on the straightaways and around turns.

- Genetic Contributions to Speed: The heritability of speed is a key consideration in breeding decisions. Studying the genetic lineage of successful racing greyhounds helps breeders identify and perpetuate the genes associated with superior speed, ensuring that each generation has the potential to excel on the track.

2. Endurance and Stamina:

- Sustained Performance: Endurance and stamina are critical for greyhounds participating in longer-distance races. Breeding for these qualities involves selecting individuals with the physiological capacity to maintain a consistent and strong pace throughout the entirety of a race, particularly in events that demand prolonged effort.

- Balancing Speed and Stamina: Achieving a balance between speed and stamina is a delicate aspect of breeding. While speed is crucial for short sprints, endurance becomes a defining factor in longer races. Breeding programs aim to produce greyhounds with a harmonious blend of these attributes to perform well across various race distances.

3. Agility and Maneuverability:

- Navigating the Racetrack: Agility and maneuverability are essential for greyhounds to navigate the twists and turns of a racetrack effectively. Breeding for these qualities involves selecting individuals with a well-coordinated and responsive musculoskeletal system, enabling precise movements and quick adjustments during races.

- Role of Skeletal Conformation: Skeletal conformation plays a significant role in agility. Breeding programs assess the structure of a greyhound's bones and joints to ensure optimal biomechanics. Proper conformation reduces the risk of injuries and enhances the greyhound's ability to execute agile maneuvers with minimal strain.

4. Focus and Determination:

- Mental Attributes: Beyond physical traits, the mental attributes of focus and determination are integral to racing success. Breeding programs consider the temperament and behavior of potential breeding pairs, aiming to perpetuate qualities such as a strong work ethic, competitiveness, and a focused demeanor during races.

- Training Adaptability: Greyhounds with a high level of focus and determination often display adaptability to training regimens. Breeding for these mental attributes contributes to producing individuals that respond well to conditioning, learn racing strategies effectively, and maintain a competitive mindset throughout their careers.

5. Health and Injury Resistance:

- Overall Health Considerations: Ethical breeding prioritizes the overall health and well-being of racing greyhounds. This includes selecting breeding pairs with a history of sound health, free from hereditary conditions that may compromise a greyhound's racing career. Genetic screenings and health assessments are integral to breeding decisions.

- Minimizing Injury Risks: Breeding programs aim to minimize the risks of injuries by selecting individuals with robust musculoskeletal systems. Genetic factors influencing bone density, joint structure, and muscle composition are assessed to reduce the susceptibility of greyhounds to injuries during training and races.

6. Adaptability to Racing Conditions:

- Performance in Varied Environments: Racing greyhounds encounter varied track conditions, including different surfaces and weather elements. Breeding for adaptability involves selecting individuals capable of performing well under diverse circumstances, ensuring that greyhounds can excel in a range of racing environments.

- Consideration of Racing Distances: Adaptability is also linked to the consideration of racing distances. Breeding programs assess the suitability of breeding pairs for specific distances, whether it be short sprints or longer races. This ensures that the offspring inherit the traits necessary for success in their intended racing events.

7. Consistency in Racing Performance:

- Reproducibility of Traits: Consistency in racing performance is a desired outcome of successful breeding programs. Breeders seek to reproduce desirable traits across generations, establishing bloodlines known for their reliability and the ability to consistently produce greyhounds with the qualities needed for success on the racetrack.

- Monitoring Bloodline Success: Breeding programs track the success of specific bloodlines over time. The performance of greyhounds from particular lineages provides valuable feedback, allowing breeders to refine their breeding strategies and identify bloodlines that consistently produce high-caliber racing greyhounds.

8. Ethical Considerations in Breeding Practices:

- Responsible Breeding Decisions: Ethical considerations in breeding extend beyond performance traits. Breeders are mindful of the ethical responsibility to prioritize the welfare of the animals they breed. This includes ensuring that breeding practices align with standards promoting the health, care, and ethical treatment of racing greyhounds.

- Balancing Tradition and Ethical Stewardship: Balancing the tradition of breeding for racing excellence with ethical stewardship is an ongoing challenge. Responsible breeding practices seek to honor the heritage of greyhound racing while adapting to evolving societal expectations and ethical considerations within the broader context of animal welfare.

Conclusion - Nurturing the Next Generation of Champions:

Desirable qualities in racing greyhounds form the foundation for nurturing the next generation of champions. By carefully selecting breeding pairs and considering the physical, temperamental, and performance attributes outlined in this chapter, breeders contribute to the ongoing legacy of greyhound racing, fostering a lineage of exceptional athletes that embody the qualities essential for success on the racetrack.

Selective Breeding Practices Over Time

The evolution of greyhound racing has been intricately tied to the practice of selective breeding, a process that has transformed the sport and shaped the characteristics of racing greyhounds. This chapter delves into the historical development and progression of selective breeding practices over time, examining the key factors, methodologies, and influential breeders that have contributed to the refinement and enhancement of greyhound bloodlines.

1. Early Days of Informal Selection:

- Origins of Greyhound Racing: In the early days of greyhound racing, the selection of breeding pairs was often an informal and decentralized process. Greyhounds were bred based on local needs, and the emphasis was on producing individuals that displayed natural speed and hunting instincts, traits essential for coursing game.

- Localized Bloodlines: Different regions developed their own localized bloodlines, reflecting the specific needs and preferences of local greyhound racing communities. These bloodlines laid the foundation for the diversity seen in the early greyhound population and contributed to the emergence of distinct regional racing styles.

2. Formalization of Breeding Practices:

- Transition to Organized Racing: As greyhound racing transitioned from informal, community-based events to organized, formalized competitions, the need for a more systematic approach to breeding became evident. The emergence of organized tracks and competitions prompted a shift towards more deliberate and strategic breeding practices.

- Influence of Organized Kennels: The establishment of organized kennels played a pivotal role in formalizing breeding practices. Kennel owners and trainers began to recognize the importance of selecting breeding pairs based on desirable racing traits, laying the groundwork for the systematic development of bloodlines.

3. Kennel Influence and Line Breeding:

- Kennel Legacy and Influence: Influential kennels emerged as key players in shaping the future of greyhound racing through their commitment to producing exceptional athletes. These kennels often developed distinct bloodlines that carried their legacy, with each generation building upon the successes of the previous.

- Introduction of Line Breeding: Line breeding, a practice that involves mating individuals within the same ancestral line, gained prominence during this period. Kennels utilized line breeding to concentrate desirable traits, creating bloodlines known for specific qualities such as speed, endurance, or agility.

4. The Role of Performance Data:

- Introduction of Performance Records: With the advancement of organized racing, the collection and analysis of performance data became a valuable tool for breeders. Keeping detailed records of individual greyhound performances allowed breeders to make informed decisions about which individuals to pair for future generations.

- Performance-Based Selection: The use of performance data shifted breeding practices towards a more performance-based selection process. Greyhounds with proven track records were often preferred as breeding stock, contributing to the refinement of bloodlines based on tangible racing success.

5. Contributions of Influential Breeders:

- Notable Breeders in Greyhound History: Throughout the history of greyhound racing, certain individuals have stood out as influential breeders who significantly impacted the sport. Their contributions, whether through the development of successful bloodlines or the introduction of innovative breeding practices, have left a lasting legacy.

- Innovation and Experimentation: Influential breeders were often innovators and experimenters, willing to push the boundaries of traditional breeding practices. Their willingness to explore new approaches, whether in terms of selection criteria or breeding methodologies, has played a crucial role in the ongoing evolution of greyhound bloodlines.

6. Technological Advancements in Breeding:

- Introduction of Genetic Testing: The integration of genetic testing into breeding practices marked a significant advancement. Breeders started utilizing genetic testing to identify specific genes associated with desirable traits, providing a more precise and scientific approach to selective breeding.

- Impact of Reproductive Technologies: Reproductive technologies, such as artificial insemination and in vitro fertilization, have also influenced breeding practices. These technologies allow breeders to overcome logistical challenges and expand their access to genetic material, contributing to the diversity and adaptability of bloodlines.

7. Challenges and Ethical Considerations:

- Balancing Tradition and Innovation: The evolution of selective breeding practices brings forth the challenge of balancing tradition with innovation. Ethical considerations arise as breeders navigate the fine line between preserving the heritage of greyhound racing and adapting to advancements that enhance the health and performance of the athletes.

- Avoiding Overemphasis on Traits: Ethical breeders strive to avoid overemphasizing certain traits to the detriment of the overall health and well-being of greyhounds. Responsible breeding practices consider a holistic approach that prioritizes the balance of physical and mental attributes, avoiding the potential pitfalls of overemphasis on specific traits.

8. The Future of Selective Breeding:

- Integration of New Technologies: The future of selective breeding in greyhound racing is likely to be influenced by ongoing advancements in technology. From more sophisticated genetic analyses to emerging tools for assessing behavioral traits, breeders will continue to integrate new technologies to refine and enhance bloodlines.

- Addressing Welfare Concerns: Ethical considerations will play an increasingly prominent role in the future of selective breeding. The greyhound racing community is likely to focus on addressing welfare concerns, including the responsible treatment of breeding animals and the ethical considerations associated with genetic selection.

Conclusion - Nurturing the Genetic Legacy:

Selective breeding practices over time have shaped the genetic legacy of greyhound racing. From the early days of informal selection to the integration of cutting-edge technologies, the evolution of bloodlines reflects a commitment to excellence and a continuous pursuit of producing greyhounds that embody the ideal combination of speed, agility, and determination on the racetrack. The ongoing journey of selective breeding remains a testament to the dedication of breeders in nurturing the genetic heritage of this remarkable and resilient breed.

Top Breeders and Kennel Lineages

The world of greyhound racing has been shaped by the dedication and expertise of top breeders and kennel lineages. This chapter explores the influential individuals and kennels that have made significant contributions to the development and refinement of greyhound bloodlines, leaving a lasting impact on the sport's history and the genetic legacy of racing greyhounds.

1. Pioneering Breeders in Greyhound Racing:

- Early Visionaries: In the early days of greyhound racing, visionaries emerged as pioneers in selective breeding. These breeders, often driven by a passion for the sport and a deep understanding of canine genetics, laid the groundwork for the systematic development of bloodlines.

- Legacy of Foundational Bloodlines: Foundational bloodlines established by early breeders became the building blocks of greyhound racing. These bloodlines, characterized by specific traits and racing abilities, set the stage for subsequent generations of greyhounds and influenced the evolution of the sport.

2. Kennels That Shaped Racing History:

- Influential Kennels: Certain kennels emerged as key players in shaping the history of greyhound racing. These kennels distinguished themselves through a commitment to excellence, producing generations of greyhounds that not only excelled on the racetrack but also contributed to the development of distinct bloodlines.

- Multi-Generational Success: The hallmark of influential kennels is often their ability to achieve success across multiple generations. Greyhounds from these kennels consistently demonstrated the desired traits, leading to the establishment of enduring bloodlines that became synonymous with racing excellence.

3. Legacy of Notable Breeders:

- Individual Contributions: Notable breeders, through their individual expertise and commitment, have left an indelible mark on greyhound racing. These individuals, whether known for their keen eye in selecting breeding pairs or innovative approaches to genetic improvement, have significantly shaped the genetic landscape of the sport.

- Introducing Innovative Practices: The legacy of notable breeders often includes the introduction of innovative breeding practices. From the strategic use of line breeding to the incorporation of cutting-edge technologies, these breeders have pushed the boundaries of traditional practices, contributing to the ongoing evolution of bloodlines.

4. Kennel Lineages and Family Traditions:

- Family-Owned Kennels: Many influential kennel lineages are characterized by a tradition of family ownership. Passed down through generations, these family-owned kennels have preserved a commitment to the sport and a dedication to maintaining and improving bloodlines.

- Transmission of Knowledge: Family-owned kennels serve as vessels of knowledge, with experienced breeders passing down insights and techniques to successive generations. This transmission of knowledge ensures the continuity of breeding practices and the preservation of the kennel's legacy.

5. Breeding for Specific Traits:

- Specialization in Traits: Top breeders and kennels often specialize in breeding for specific traits. Whether it be an emphasis on speed, agility, or endurance, these breeders strategically select pairs to enhance and concentrate the desired qualities, contributing to the development of specialized bloodlines.

- Diversification of Bloodlines: While specialization is common, top breeders also recognize the importance of diversification within bloodlines. The ability to adapt to changing racing conditions and requirements necessitates a balance between concentrating desirable traits and maintaining genetic diversity.

6. Modern Innovations in Breeding:

- Technological Advancements: Modern top breeders embrace technological advancements in breeding practices. From genetic testing to reproductive technologies, these breeders leverage scientific tools to make informed decisions, identify desirable traits, and ensure the health and well-being of breeding animals.

- Data-Driven Decision-Making: The integration of data-driven decision-making has become a hallmark of modern breeding practices. Breeders analyze performance data, genetic markers, and health records to make strategic decisions that contribute to the continued improvement of bloodlines.

7. Global Influence of Top Breeders:

- International Impact: The influence of top breeders extends beyond regional boundaries, with some gaining international recognition for their contributions. Breeders who have achieved success on a global scale have played a crucial role in disseminating knowledge, improving bloodlines worldwide, and fostering collaboration within the global greyhound racing community.

- Exchange of Breeding Practices: International collaboration has facilitated the exchange of breeding practices and methodologies. This exchange contributes to a shared pool of knowledge, allowing breeders from different regions to benefit from diverse perspectives and approaches to breeding.

8. Challenges and Ethical Considerations:

- Ethical Responsibilities of Top Breeders: Top breeders bear ethical responsibilities to ensure the welfare of the animals they breed. This includes considerations such as responsible breeding practices, proper care for breeding animals, and a commitment to addressing ethical concerns within the greyhound racing community.

- Navigating Challenges: As stewards of the sport, top breeders navigate challenges such as changing public perceptions, evolving legislative landscapes, and heightened scrutiny on animal welfare. Ethical and responsible breeding practices are integral to addressing these challenges and sustaining the long-term viability of greyhound racing.

Conclusion - Shaping the Future of Greyhound Racing:

Top breeders and kennel lineages play a pivotal role in shaping the future of greyhound racing. Their expertise, dedication, and commitment to excellence contribute not only to the ongoing success of individual greyhounds but also to the preservation and evolution of bloodlines that define the sport. As stewards of the genetic legacy, top breeders continue to shape the trajectory of greyhound racing, ensuring its resilience and adaptability in the face of a changing landscape.

Contribution of Genetics vs. Training

The perennial debate in greyhound racing revolves around the relative contributions of genetics and training to the success of racing greyhounds. This chapter delves into the intricate interplay between a greyhound's genetic makeup and the training it undergoes, exploring how both elements shape the performance and capabilities of these remarkable athletes on the racetrack.

1. The Genetic Blueprint of Racing Greyhounds:

- Inherited Traits and Characteristics: The genetic foundation of racing greyhounds dictates a range of inherited traits and characteristics. These include physical attributes such as speed, agility, endurance, as well as behavioral traits like temperament and willingness to chase the lure.

- Understanding Canine Genetics: To comprehend the contribution of genetics, it is essential to understand the basics of canine genetics. The inheritance of genes from parent to offspring plays a critical role in determining the inherent abilities and predispositions of racing greyhounds.

2. Selective Breeding and Genetic Enhancement:

- Purposeful Breeding for Traits: Selective breeding practices are specifically designed to enhance desirable traits in racing greyhounds. Breeders aim to concentrate genes associated with speed, stamina, and other essential racing attributes, contributing to the development of bloodlines known for their racing prowess.

- Impact of Line Breeding: Line breeding, a technique used to intensify specific genetic traits within a bloodline, plays a crucial role. The concentrated genetic material resulting from line breeding contributes to the transmission of desirable traits from one generation to the next.

3. Genetic Diversity and Adaptability:

- Balancing Genetic Diversity: While concentrated genetic traits are desirable, maintaining a balance of genetic diversity is crucial for the overall health and adaptability of the greyhound population. Genetic diversity helps mitigate the risk of inherited disorders and ensures a resilient and versatile breed.

- Adaptability to Racing Conditions: Genetic diversity contributes to the adaptability of greyhounds to various racing conditions. A diverse genetic pool allows for the development of greyhounds with the flexibility to excel on different track surfaces, in varying climates, and under diverse competition scenarios.

4. Training as a Shaping Force:

- Training's Role in Development: Training is a dynamic force that shapes the potential encoded in a greyhound's genetic makeup. It influences physical fitness, muscle development, and the honing of racing skills. A well-structured training regimen is essential for unlocking a greyhound's full potential.

- Mental and Physical Conditioning: Training extends beyond physical conditioning to include mental preparedness. Greyhounds undergo training to enhance their focus, discipline, and ability to respond to cues, crucial elements for success on the racetrack.

5. Nature vs. Nurture Debate:

- Genetic Predisposition vs. Environmental Influence: The age-old debate of nature versus nurture finds resonance in greyhound racing. While genetics provide the initial blueprint, environmental factors, including training methods, nutrition, and living conditions, contribute significantly to the actualization of a greyhound's potential.

- Identifying Genetic Potential: Trainers use early indicators, such as a greyhound's pedigree and lineage, to gauge its genetic potential. This information guides trainers in tailoring training programs that align with the inherent strengths and weaknesses associated with a particular bloodline.

6. The Role of Epigenetics:

- Understanding Epigenetic Factors: Epigenetics, the study of changes in gene function that do not involve alterations to the underlying DNA sequence, plays a role in the interaction between genetics and training. Environmental factors, including training stimuli, can influence gene expression and impact a greyhound's performance.

- Epigenetic Adaptations to Training: Training-induced adaptations at the epigenetic level highlight the dynamic nature of the interplay between genetics and training. These adaptations can influence a greyhound's response to specific training techniques and contribute to its overall racing abilities.

7. Genetic Limitations and Training Optimization:

- Acknowledging Genetic Limitations: Every greyhound has inherent genetic limitations. While selective breeding aims to enhance desirable traits, acknowledging and understanding these limitations is crucial for realistic expectations and effective training strategies.

- Optimizing Training for Individual Differences: Trainers must tailor their approaches to account for individual variations in genetic predispositions. Recognizing the unique strengths and weaknesses of each greyhound allows trainers to optimize training methods for maximum effectiveness.

8. The Symbiosis of Genetics and Training:

- Complementary Forces: Ultimately, the success of a racing greyhound is the result of the symbiotic relationship between genetics and training. Genetics provide the foundation and potential, while training acts as the sculptor, shaping and refining that potential into a finely tuned racing athlete.

- Continuous Interaction: The interaction between genetics and training is not a one-time event but a continuous process throughout a greyhound's racing career. As the greyhound matures and gains experience, the ongoing interplay between genetics and training continues to influence its performance.

Conclusion - Nurturing Potential for Racing Excellence:

In the realm of greyhound racing, the contribution of genetics versus training is not a binary equation but a nuanced interplay. Successful breeding practices set the stage for potential, and training acts as the catalyst, unlocking and refining that potential. Embracing the complexity of this relationship is essential for breeders, trainers, and enthusiasts alike, as they collectively nurture the genetic and trained capabilities that define the excellence of racing greyhounds.

Future of Selective Breeding in the Sport

As greyhound racing navigates the currents of modernity, the future of the sport hinges on the trajectory of selective breeding. This chapter delves into the evolving landscape of greyhound breeding, exploring the challenges, innovations, and ethical considerations that will shape the genetic destinies of racing greyhounds in the years to come.

1. Technological Advancements in Selective Breeding:

- Genetic Mapping and Sequencing: The future of selective breeding is deeply intertwined with advancements in genetic mapping and sequencing technologies. These tools offer unprecedented insights into the greyhound genome, enabling breeders to identify and understand the genetic markers associated with racing prowess.

- Precision Breeding Techniques: Emerging techniques in precision breeding, facilitated by technologies like CRISPR-Cas9, hold the potential to precisely edit or modify specific genes. While in its infancy and ethically complex, this technology may offer avenues for targeted improvements in desirable racing traits.

2. Data-Driven Decision-Making:

- Integration of Performance Data: The future of selective breeding will see an increased reliance on data-driven decision-making. Breeders will leverage comprehensive performance data, including race results, health records, and genetic markers, to inform breeding choices and optimize the potential for racing success.

- Machine Learning Applications: Machine learning algorithms will play a role in analyzing vast datasets, identifying patterns, and predicting breeding outcomes. This integration of artificial intelligence into breeding practices has the potential to refine and enhance the precision of selective breeding.

3. Ethical Considerations and Animal Welfare:

- Enhanced Ethical Oversight: As technology evolves, ethical considerations in selective breeding will come to the forefront. The future will likely witness an enhanced focus on ethical oversight, ensuring that breeding practices align with the welfare of the animals and address concerns related to genetic diversity and hereditary health issues.

- Transparency in Breeding Practices: Breeders will face increasing expectations for transparency in their practices. The future of selective breeding will involve open communication about breeding goals, methods, and outcomes, fostering a culture of accountability within the greyhound racing community.

4. Balancing Specialization and Diversity:

- Maintaining Genetic Diversity: While specialization in desirable traits is essential, the future of selective breeding will recognize the importance of maintaining genetic diversity. Balancing specialization with diversity is crucial for the long-term health and adaptability of the greyhound population.

- Adaptability to Changing Conditions: The unpredictable nature of racing conditions demands a breed that can adapt. The future of breeding will strive to produce greyhounds with the flexibility to excel across diverse tracks, climates, and competition scenarios.

5. Global Collaboration and Knowledge Exchange:

- International Collaboration: The future of selective breeding will witness increased collaboration among breeders on a global scale. Sharing knowledge, experiences, and genetic resources will contribute to a more interconnected community, fostering a collective effort to enhance the genetic potential of racing greyhounds.

- Cross-Border Genetic Contributions: International collaboration will extend beyond knowledge exchange to include cross-border genetic contributions. Breeders may explore the introduction of genetic material from diverse regional populations to enhance genetic diversity and introduce novel racing traits.

6. Community Engagement and Public Perception:

- Education and Outreach Programs: The future of selective breeding will involve proactive education and outreach programs to engage the broader community. Breeders will play a role in demystifying the breeding process, dispelling myths, and fostering a better understanding of the ethical considerations inherent in greyhound breeding.

- Addressing Public Concerns: Acknowledging and addressing public concerns related to greyhound breeding practices will be paramount. Breeders will engage in open dialogues with the public, addressing questions about animal welfare, ethical breeding, and the responsible stewardship of racing greyhounds.

7. Environmental Considerations and Sustainability:

- Climate-Adaptive Breeding: Climate change may influence racing conditions, necessitating a future-oriented approach to breeding. Breeders may explore climate-adaptive breeding practices to ensure that greyhounds remain well-suited to evolving environmental conditions.

- Sustainable Breeding Practices: Sustainable breeding practices will be a focal point in the future of greyhound breeding. Striking a balance between breeding for racing performance and the overall sustainability of the breed will be essential for the long-term viability of greyhound racing.

8. Regulatory Frameworks and Industry Standards:

- Evolution of Regulations: The future will likely witness the evolution of regulatory frameworks governing greyhound breeding. Regulatory bodies may adapt to incorporate advancements in technology, ethical standards, and public expectations, ensuring that breeding practices align with the broader values of society.

- Industry-Led Standards: The greyhound racing industry itself will play a pivotal role in setting and upholding breeding standards. Industry-led initiatives may establish guidelines for responsible breeding, addressing welfare concerns, and promoting the continued improvement of racing bloodlines.

Conclusion - Nurturing the Genetic Legacy:

The future of selective breeding in greyhound racing is a dynamic and multifaceted journey. It involves the responsible integration of cutting-edge technologies, a commitment to ethical considerations, and a dedication to preserving the genetic legacy of racing greyhounds. As stewards of this remarkable breed, breeders will navigate the complexities of the evolving landscape, striving to enhance the potential and well-being of future generations of racing greyhounds.

Chapter 7: Owners, Trainers, and Handlers
Leading Owners and Racing Syndicates

In the intricate world of greyhound racing, the role of owners and racing syndicates is pivotal. This chapter unravels the stories of those who invest their passion, resources, and strategic acumen into the sport. From individual owners to powerful racing syndicates, the chapter explores the dynamics of ownership, the thrill of competition, and the pursuit of excellence on the racetrack.

1. The Essence of Ownership:

- Investment Beyond Finances: Being an owner in the world of greyhound racing is more than a financial investment; it's a commitment of heart and soul. Owners share a profound connection with their greyhounds, often viewing them as not just athletes but as valued companions and members of the family.

- Passion and Commitment: Leading owners are distinguished by their unwavering passion for the sport. Their commitment extends beyond the race itself, encompassing the well-being of their greyhounds, involvement in the racing community, and a dedication to upholding the integrity of the sport.

2. Racing Syndicates:

- Collaborative Ownership Model: Racing syndicates represent a collaborative ownership model where a group of individuals come together to share ownership of a greyhound. This approach allows enthusiasts to pool resources, share the excitement of ownership, and participate in the highs and lows of competitive racing.

- Diversity of Syndicate Structures: Racing syndicates vary in structure, ranging from small groups of friends to larger, professionally managed entities. The chapter explores the diverse landscape of racing syndicates, highlighting their impact on the accessibility and democratization of ownership within the sport.

3. Profiles of Leading Owners:

- Trailblazers in Greyhound Ownership: The chapter delves into the stories of leading owners who have left an indelible mark on the sport. From those who have achieved success through strategic breeding to others whose commitment to their greyhounds has become legendary, these profiles offer insights into the diverse paths to ownership excellence.

- The Impact of Owners on the Sport: Leading owners not only contribute to the competitive landscape but also shape the sport's narrative. Their choices, successes, and even challenges influence the direction of greyhound racing, making them key players in the broader ecosystem of the sport.

4. Racing Syndicate Success Stories:

- Collective Achievements: Success stories of racing syndicates showcase the power of collective efforts. Whether through astute selection of breeding pairs, strategic race planning, or the collaborative expertise of syndicate members, these narratives illustrate the achievements that can arise from shared ownership.

- Building a Sense of Community: Racing syndicates foster a sense of community among members. The chapter explores how syndicates create a shared experience, building connections among individuals who may have otherwise never crossed paths, all united by a common love for greyhound racing.

5. Challenges of Ownership and Syndication:

- Financial Considerations: Owning and managing racing greyhounds come with financial considerations. The chapter discusses the economic aspects of ownership, exploring how owners and syndicates navigate costs, investments, and the potential for financial returns in a sport driven by passion.

- Navigating Competition and Expectations: Leading owners and racing syndicates face the challenge of navigating the competitive landscape and managing expectations. The chapter delves into the strategies employed by successful owners to stay ahead in a field where variables are numerous and outcomes unpredictable.

6. Strategic Decision-Making:

- Breeding and Acquisition Choices: The strategic decisions of owners, whether in breeding selections or acquiring racing greyhounds, significantly impact their chances of success. The chapter explores the decision-making processes of leading owners and syndicates, shedding light on the blend of intuition, data analysis, and experience that guides their choices.

- Trusting the Expertise of Trainers: Successful owners recognize the importance of collaboration with trainers. The relationship between owners and trainers is a symbiotic one, where trust and communication are paramount. The chapter explores how leading owners build and maintain these partnerships to optimize the performance of their greyhounds.

7. The Emotional Landscape of Ownership:

- Joy and Heartbreak: The emotional rollercoaster of greyhound ownership is explored, encompassing the jubilation of victory and the heartbreak of defeat. Owners invest not only in the pursuit of success but also in the emotional highs and lows that come with the territory.

- The Bond Between Owners and Greyhounds: Leading owners often speak of the deep bond they share with their greyhounds. This section explores the profound connections that develop between owners and their racing companions, highlighting the unique and enduring nature of these relationships.

8. The Future of Ownership and Syndication:

- Innovations in Ownership Models: The future of greyhound ownership may witness innovations in ownership models. From blockchain-based ownership structures to virtual syndicates, the chapter speculates on potential developments that could reshape how individuals and groups engage with the sport.

- Community Engagement Initiatives: Owners and syndicates will likely play an active role in community engagement initiatives. The chapter explores how leading figures in ownership may contribute to initiatives that promote the sport, engage fans, and foster a sense of belonging within the greyhound racing community.

Conclusion - Owners as Custodians of the Sport:

In the grand tapestry of greyhound racing, owners and racing syndicates emerge not only as stakeholders but as custodians of the sport's legacy. Their stories, triumphs, and challenges weave into the fabric of greyhound racing, shaping its narrative and ensuring that the passion for the sport endures for generations to come.

Famous Trainers and Their Methods

Within the dynamic world of greyhound racing, trainers stand as the architects of success, shaping the athletic prowess and competitive spirit of their canine charges. This chapter delves into the profiles of renowned trainers whose methods have left an indelible mark on the sport. From time-tested training regimens to innovative approaches, the narratives unfold the art and science behind the success of these iconic figures.

1. The Craftsmanship of Training:

- The Trainer's Crucial Role: Trainers play a pivotal role in the development of racing greyhounds. This section introduces the significance of a trainer's role, emphasizing their influence on a greyhound's physical conditioning, mental acuity, and overall preparedness for the rigors of the racetrack.

- Balancing Science and Intuition: Successful trainers master the delicate balance between scientific principles and intuitive understanding. Their methods encompass a fusion of empirical knowledge, behavioral psychology, and a deep connection with their greyhounds, creating a holistic approach to training.

2. Profiles of Famous Trainers:

- Legendary Figures in Greyhound Training: The chapter profiles legendary trainers whose names resonate through the history of greyhound racing. From pioneers who laid the foundations to modern maestros, each profile provides insights into the trainer's journey, achievements, and the training philosophies that set them apart.

- Diversity in Training Approaches: Famous trainers often showcase a diverse range of training approaches. Some may emphasize traditional methods rooted in decades of experience, while others may adopt innovative techniques aligned with contemporary understanding of animal behavior and performance optimization.

3. Training Philosophies and Principles:

- Fitness and Conditioning: A core aspect of greyhound training revolves around fitness and conditioning. Famous trainers focus on developing a greyhound's strength, speed, and endurance through tailored exercise routines, ensuring peak physical performance on race day.

- Mental Preparedness: Beyond physical prowess, mental preparedness is a cornerstone of successful greyhound training. Trainers employ techniques to build focus, resilience, and a positive attitude in their charges, factors that can significantly impact a greyhound's performance under the pressures of competition.

4. Nutrition and Health Management:

- Tailored Nutrition Plans: Famous trainers understand the importance of nutrition in a greyhound's performance. They collaborate with veterinarians and nutritionists to design tailored meal plans that provide the necessary nutrients for optimal health, energy levels, and recovery.

- Health Monitoring and Preventive Care: A comprehensive approach to training includes diligent health monitoring and preventive care. Trainers implement strategies to identify and address potential health issues before they impact performance, ensuring that greyhounds are in peak condition throughout their racing careers.

5. Building Relationships with Greyhounds:

- Trust and Bonding: Successful trainers forge deep bonds of trust and understanding with their greyhounds. This section explores how trainers establish positive relationships, recognizing the unique personalities of each greyhound and tailoring their training methods to suit individual needs.

- Communication and Body Language: The art of training extends to effective communication. Trainers adeptly interpret and respond to the subtle cues and body language of their greyhounds, fostering a communication channel that enhances the training experience and strengthens the human-canine connection.

6. Adaptability and Innovation:

- Adapting to Individual Needs: The most effective trainers demonstrate adaptability in their methods, recognizing that each greyhound is a unique athlete with distinct strengths and challenges. They adjust training regimens based on individual needs, maximizing the potential for success.

- Incorporating Technological Innovations: Embracing technological advancements, some trainers integrate tools like GPS tracking, heart rate monitors, and data analytics into their training programs. This infusion of technology allows for precise monitoring and optimization of training routines.

7. Success Stories and Career Highlights:

- Landmark Achievements: The chapter highlights the landmark achievements of famous trainers, from notable race victories to records broken. Each success story provides a glimpse into the culmination of meticulous training, strategic planning, and the enduring partnership between trainers and their greyhounds.

- Legacy Beyond the Racetrack: The impact of famous trainers extends beyond the immediate glory of race wins. Their legacy is often marked by the continued success of greyhounds they've trained, the development of future trainers influenced by their methods, and a lasting imprint on the sport itself.

8. Challenges and Triumphs:

- Navigating Challenges: Even the most celebrated trainers face challenges, whether in the form of injuries, unexpected setbacks, or the evolving landscape of the racing industry. This section explores how famous trainers navigate challenges and adapt their methods to ensure sustained success.

- Triumphs in Adversity: Triumphs in the face of adversity are emblematic of a trainer's resilience and expertise. The chapter presents instances where trainers have overcome obstacles, showcasing the determination and skill that characterize the best in the field.

Conclusion - The Enduring Impact of Trainers:

Famous trainers leave an enduring impact on greyhound racing, shaping the sport's narrative through their dedication, expertise, and transformative methods. Their influence extends far beyond the racetrack, resonating in the achievements of the greyhounds they've trained and the continued evolution of training practices within the dynamic world of greyhound racing.

Handlers and Their Relationships with Dogs

In the intricate dance of greyhound racing, handlers play a crucial role as the bridge between the racing greyhounds and their owners and trainers. This chapter delves into the world of handlers, exploring the depth of their relationships with the dogs under their care. From the day-to-day routines to the emotional bonds formed in the racing kennels, the narratives unfold the unique dynamics that define the handler-dog connection.

1. The Significance of Handlers:

- Link Between Kennel and Racetrack: Handlers serve as the vital link between the controlled environment of the kennel and the electrifying atmosphere of the racetrack. Their responsibilities extend beyond routine care to include preparing greyhounds for races, ensuring their well-being, and interpreting their needs to the wider team.

- Nurturing the Human-Canine Bond: Handlers play a central role in nurturing the human-canine bond. This section introduces the multifaceted nature of handler responsibilities, encompassing physical care, emotional support, and the building of trust with racing greyhounds.

2. Daily Routines and Care:

- Feeding and Exercise Regimens: Handlers are entrusted with the daily care of racing greyhounds, including adhering to carefully curated feeding plans and exercise regimens. This section explores the meticulous routines handlers follow to maintain the health, fitness, and well-being of their charges.

- Monitoring Health and Behavior: The close relationship between handlers and greyhounds enables them to be attuned to subtle changes in behavior and health. Handlers act as the first line of defense against potential issues, monitoring for signs of discomfort, illness, or any changes that may impact a greyhound's readiness for racing.

3. Race Day Preparation:

- Pre-Race Rituals: Race day preparation is a collaborative effort between trainers and handlers. Handlers engage in pre-race rituals designed to mentally and physically prepare the greyhounds for the upcoming competition. This section details the routines and practices employed to optimize a greyhound's readiness.

- Calm and Focus Techniques: Handlers play a crucial role in maintaining a greyhound's calm and focused demeanor on race day. Techniques such as massage, positive reinforcement, and calming rituals are explored, shedding light on the methods used to channel a greyhound's energy into a focused and competitive state.

4. Building Trust and Understanding:

- Establishing Trustful Relationships: Trust is the foundation of the handler-dog relationship. This section delves into how handlers establish and nurture trustful connections with their greyhounds, emphasizing the importance of mutual understanding and communication in the racing kennel environment.

- Recognizing Individual Personalities: Each greyhound has a distinct personality, and handlers become adept at recognizing and understanding these individual traits. The chapter explores how handlers tailor their approaches to suit the unique needs and preferences of each dog, fostering a personalized and supportive environment.

5. Communication and Body Language:

- Non-Verbal Communication: Handlers communicate with greyhounds through nuanced non-verbal cues and body language. This section delves into the subtleties of handler-dog communication, highlighting the importance of a shared language that transcends words and enhances the connection between the two.

- Interpreting Greyhound Signals: Successful handlers become proficient in interpreting the signals and cues provided by greyhounds. Understanding the nuances of a wagging tail, a certain posture, or a specific bark allows handlers to respond appropriately, ensuring the comfort and well-being of their canine companions.

6. Emotional Support and Comfort:

- Coping with Stress and Anxiety: Racing greyhounds, like any athletes, may experience stress and anxiety. Handlers provide emotional support, offering comfort and reassurance to alleviate any pre-race nerves. This section explores the strategies employed by handlers to create a positive and calming environment.

- Building Emotional Bonds: The emotional bonds formed between handlers and greyhounds transcend the functional aspects of their relationship. Handlers often become steadfast companions to the dogs, providing a source of emotional security and companionship within the racing kennel.

7. Challenges and Rewards of Handling:

- Navigating Challenges: Handlers encounter various challenges, from handling injuries and setbacks to managing the pressures of race day. This section explores how experienced handlers navigate these challenges, drawing on their expertise and the relationships they've cultivated with their greyhounds.

- The Rewards of the Connection: The rewards of handling extend beyond the racetrack. Handlers find fulfillment in witnessing the success of the greyhounds they've cared for, in the bonds formed, and in the unique joys that come from being an integral part of the racing community.

8. Evolving Role of Handlers:

- Adapting to Changing Dynamics: The role of handlers evolves in tandem with changes in the racing industry, technology, and societal attitudes towards animal welfare. This section explores how handlers adapt to these dynamics, embracing innovations while maintaining the core principles of their craft.

- Advocacy for Greyhound Well-Being: Handlers often become advocates for greyhound welfare. The chapter discusses how handlers, through their daily interactions and understanding of the dogs, contribute to broader conversations about the well-being and ethical treatment of racing greyhounds.

Conclusion - The Heartbeat of the Kennel:

Handlers stand as the heartbeat of the racing kennel, embodying the dedication, skill, and compassion essential to the well-being and success of racing greyhounds. Their relationships with the dogs extend far beyond the functional aspects of their duties, shaping the emotional landscape of the racing community and leaving an enduring impact on the sport.

Rags to Riches Stories of Success

Amidst the competitive realm of greyhound racing, tales of triumph often emerge from humble beginnings. This chapter delves into the inspirational narratives of individuals who, against the odds, rose from obscurity to achieve prominence as owners, trainers, or handlers within the world of greyhound racing. These rags-to-riches stories not only underscore the resilience and determination of those involved but also offer a glimpse into the transformative power of passion and dedication in the pursuit of success.

1. The Journey from Humble Beginnings:

- Forging Paths from the Ground Up: Rags-to-riches stories often commence with individuals who entered the world of greyhound racing with limited resources but boundless enthusiasm. This section explores the early days of these individuals, highlighting the challenges they faced and the initial steps taken to establish themselves in the industry.

- Passion Ignites the Spark: Passion for greyhounds and the sport itself serves as the driving force behind many success stories. The chapter delves into the transformative power of passion, examining how individuals discovered their love for greyhound racing and turned it into a driving force for personal and professional growth.

2. Owners Who Defied the Odds:

- From Enthusiasts to Owners: Some owners started as enthusiasts, drawn to the excitement and beauty of greyhound racing. This section explores how these individuals transitioned from spectators to owners, often overcoming financial constraints and societal expectations to pursue their dreams in the racing industry.

- Investment and Risk: Rags-to-riches stories in ownership involve risk and investment. The chapter discusses how these individuals navigated the financial challenges associated with acquiring, caring for, and racing greyhounds, showcasing the calculated risks that ultimately led to success.

3. Trainers' Unlikely Journeys:

- Learning the Ropes: Aspiring trainers with modest backgrounds often embark on journeys of self-discovery and education. This section explores how individuals learned the intricacies of greyhound training, drawing on mentors, hands-on experience, and a genuine love for the sport.

- Building Kennels from Scratch: Rags-to-riches stories among trainers frequently involve the establishment of kennels from scratch. The chapter details the challenges faced by trainers in acquiring facilities, assembling teams, and developing the infrastructure necessary for successful greyhound training operations.

4. Handlers Overcoming Adversity:

- From Kennel Assistants to Handlers: Handlers often rise from humble positions as kennel assistants or caretakers. This section explores the journeys of those who transitioned from behind-the-scenes roles to becoming integral figures on race days, showcasing the determination and hard work that paved their paths.

- Skill Development and Training: Rags-to-riches stories among handlers highlight the development of essential skills. The chapter examines how individuals honed their handling techniques, built connections with greyhounds, and transformed their roles into key components of successful racing teams.

5. Defying Stereotypes and Breaking Barriers:

- Gender and Diversity Challenges: Some rags-to-riches stories involve individuals breaking through gender or diversity barriers within the traditionally male-dominated industry. The chapter explores how these trailblazers defied stereotypes and paved the way for increased inclusivity within greyhound racing.

- Elevating the Sport through Diversity: The impact of diverse voices within greyhound racing goes beyond individual success. This section discusses how individuals from varied backgrounds contribute to the richness and vibrancy of the sport, bringing new perspectives and approaches that benefit the industry as a whole.

6. Achievements and Recognition:

- Turning Heads with Success: Rags-to-riches stories gain prominence as individuals achieve notable successes within the racing community. The chapter highlights key achievements, such as significant race victories, the development of champion greyhounds, or the establishment of kennels that become forces to be reckoned with.

- Recognition within the Racing Community: Success stories often garner recognition and respect from peers within the racing community. The chapter explores how individuals who once faced skepticism or doubts earned the admiration and acknowledgment of their colleagues, solidifying their places as influential figures in the sport.

7. Paying It Forward:

- Mentorship and Support: Many who have risen from humble beginnings express a commitment to giving back. This section delves into how successful owners, trainers, and handlers become mentors and sources of support for the next generation, fostering a cycle of growth and empowerment within the greyhound racing community.

- Community Engagement and Advocacy: Rags-to-riches stories often extend beyond personal success to encompass community engagement and advocacy. The chapter explores how individuals use their platforms to advocate for the welfare of greyhounds, contribute to industry improvements, and engage with broader issues affecting the sport.

Conclusion - Inspiring the Next Generation:

Rags-to-riches stories within greyhound racing inspire not only through individual achievements but also by embodying the spirit of resilience and determination that fuels the industry's growth. These narratives serve as beacons of inspiration for aspiring owners, trainers, handlers, and enthusiasts, underscoring the limitless possibilities that arise from a genuine passion for the sport and an unwavering commitment to success.

Rising Personalities to Watch

In the ever-evolving landscape of greyhound racing, new stars emerge, bringing fresh perspectives, innovative approaches, and a passion for the sport. This chapter is dedicated to spotlighting the rising personalities within the world of greyhound racing—individuals who are making waves, challenging norms, and shaping the future of the industry. From owners with a keen eye for talent to trainers employing cutting-edge techniques and handlers exhibiting exceptional skills, these rising personalities exemplify the dynamism and potential that propel greyhound racing forward.

1. Visionary Owners with a Knack for Talent:

- Spotlight on Emerging Owners: This section introduces owners who are gaining recognition for their strategic vision, keen instincts, and commitment to elevating the caliber of racing greyhounds. It explores their backgrounds, motivations, and the impact they are making on the competitive landscape.

- Investment in Quality Bloodlines: Rising owners often distinguish themselves by their investments in quality bloodlines. The chapter delves into how these individuals strategically select and acquire greyhounds with the potential for greatness, contributing to the enhancement of racing pedigrees.

2. Trailblazing Trainers Implementing Innovation:

- Innovative Training Techniques: The spotlight turns to trainers who are at the forefront of innovation in greyhound training. This section explores how these individuals integrate technology, sports science, and unconventional methods to optimize training regimens, ensuring that their greyhounds are not only competitive but also at the forefront of athletic development.

- Balancing Tradition and Innovation: Rising trainers navigate the delicate balance between traditional methods and modern approaches. The chapter discusses how these individuals draw from time-tested techniques while incorporating contemporary advancements, fostering a harmonious blend that caters to the individual needs of their greyhounds.

3. Exceptional Handlers Crafting Success Stories:

- Skillful Handling on the Rise: Handlers who are gaining prominence for their exceptional skills take center stage in this section. It explores the nuances of their techniques, the depth of their connections with greyhounds, and the pivotal role they play in the overall success of racing teams.

- Adapting to Evolving Dynamics: The racing environment is dynamic, and rising handlers showcase adaptability. The chapter discusses how these individuals navigate changes in the industry, from evolving race formats to advancements in equipment and technology, and tailor their handling approaches accordingly.

4. Multi-Faceted Personalities Driving Change:

- Owners with Trainer Backgrounds: A rising trend in greyhound racing involves individuals who transition from successful careers as trainers to become influential owners. This section explores their unique perspectives, the insights they bring to ownership, and the ways in which their dual roles contribute to the overall success of their racing operations.

- Handlers Taking on Training Roles: Another intriguing dynamic is the emergence of handlers who expand their roles to encompass aspects of training. The chapter delves into how these multi-faceted individuals leverage their intimate knowledge of greyhounds to contribute to training strategies and enhance the overall performance of their teams.

5. Rising Stars Embracing Advocacy:

- Championing Welfare and Ethical Practices: Some rising personalities go beyond their roles in racing and actively engage in advocacy for the welfare of greyhounds. This section explores how these individuals use their platforms to champion ethical practices, promote responsible breeding, and contribute to the ongoing dialogue surrounding the well-being of racing greyhounds.

- Engaging with the Racing Community: Rising personalities often recognize the importance of community engagement. The chapter discusses how these individuals foster connections within the racing community, building networks that support the exchange of knowledge, ideas, and collaborative efforts to enhance the overall experience of greyhound racing.

6. Challenges and Triumphs of Rising Personalities:

- Navigating Industry Challenges: Rising personalities inevitably face challenges as they ascend within the racing hierarchy. This section examines the obstacles they encounter, from financial constraints to industry skepticism, and how they navigate these challenges to carve out their places as influential figures.

- Celebrating Triumphs and Milestones: Despite the hurdles, rising personalities achieve significant milestones. The chapter highlights their triumphs, whether in the form of notable race victories, the development of champion greyhounds, or the establishment of kennels and operations that become synonymous with success.

7. The Future Landscape:

- Shaping the Future of Greyhound Racing: The chapter concludes by exploring how these rising personalities are contributing to shaping the future of greyhound racing. Whether through innovations in training, strategic ownership, or advocacy efforts, these individuals play a pivotal role in ensuring the continued growth, sustainability, and positive evolution of the sport.

Conclusion - A Tapestry of Talent:

Rising personalities within greyhound racing collectively form a tapestry of talent, diversity, and passion that enriches the sport's narrative. Their stories not only inspire but also serve as a testament to the dynamic nature of greyhound racing, where the contributions of emerging individuals are instrumental in propelling the industry into an exciting and promising future.

Chapter 8: The Business of Dog Racing
Economics of the Racing Industry

The greyhound racing industry is not only a dynamic sport but also a complex business ecosystem with multifaceted economic dimensions. This chapter explores the intricate economics that underpin the world of dog racing, from revenue streams to operational costs, shedding light on the financial intricacies that contribute to the industry's vitality and sustainability.

1. Revenue Streams:

- Betting as the Primary Driver: At the heart of the greyhound racing industry's economic structure is betting. This section delves into the significance of wagering as the primary revenue driver, examining the various forms of betting, including on-site, off-site, and online platforms.

- Gate Receipts and Admission Fees: In addition to betting, gate receipts and admission fees form essential components of the industry's revenue streams. The chapter explores how tracks generate income from spectators attending races, special events, and other activities hosted at racing venues.

- Media Rights and Broadcasting Deals: The broadcasting of greyhound races, both on television and online platforms, contributes significantly to the industry's financial landscape. This section examines the role of media rights and broadcasting deals, exploring how partnerships with media outlets enhance the sport's visibility and financial standing.

2. Operational Costs:

- Care and Maintenance of Greyhounds: A substantial portion of the industry's expenses is dedicated to the care and maintenance of racing greyhounds. This section delves into the costs associated with breeding, feeding, veterinary care, and overall welfare, highlighting the industry's commitment to the well-being of its canine athletes.

- Infrastructure and Track Maintenance: Greyhound tracks are critical assets for the industry, requiring ongoing maintenance and infrastructure development. The chapter explores the operational costs associated with track facilities, including renovations, safety enhancements, and technological advancements.

- Personnel and Training Expenses: The human element is integral to the industry's operations, from trainers and handlers to administrative staff. This section examines the costs related to personnel, training programs, and the professional development of individuals involved in various capacities within the racing community.

3. Prize Pools and Incentives:

- Distribution of Prize Money: The distribution of prize money plays a crucial role in attracting top-tier competitors and maintaining a competitive racing environment. This part of the chapter explores how prize pools are structured, including the allocation of winnings to owners, trainers, handlers, and other key contributors.

- Incentives for Excellence: Incentive programs are designed to reward exceptional performances and encourage participant engagement. The chapter discusses how industry stakeholders implement incentive schemes, such as bonuses for achieving milestones or excelling in prestigious races, to enhance the competitive spirit and overall quality of racing.

4. Sponsorship and Corporate Partnerships:

- Attracting Corporate Sponsorship: Corporate sponsorship and partnerships with businesses from various industries provide additional financial support to the greyhound racing ecosystem. This section explores how tracks, events, and racing organizations attract and maintain partnerships with sponsors, fostering mutually beneficial relationships.

- Branding and Marketing Initiatives: Effective branding and marketing are vital for attracting sponsors and enhancing the industry's commercial appeal. The chapter examines how the racing community leverages branding initiatives, promotional events, and marketing strategies to expand its reach and attract corporate support.

5. Regulatory Costs and Compliance:

- Compliance with Regulatory Standards: Adherence to regulatory standards is imperative for the sustainability and legitimacy of the industry. This section discusses the costs associated with complying with regulations related to animal welfare, anti-doping measures, and overall industry oversight.

- Investment in Responsible Gaming Programs: As part of regulatory compliance, the industry invests in responsible gaming programs to address concerns related to gambling addiction and promote ethical betting practices. The chapter explores the costs associated with these initiatives and their impact on the industry's social responsibility.

6. Economic Impact on Local Communities:

- Job Creation and Local Employment: Greyhound racing contributes significantly to local economies by generating employment opportunities. This section explores how the industry creates jobs, from kennel staff and trainers to administrative roles, thereby bolstering economic activity in racing communities.

- Tourism and Ancillary Services: Racing events attract tourists and spectators, leading to increased demand for ancillary services such as hospitality, accommodations, and local businesses. The chapter examines the broader economic impact of greyhound racing on the communities surrounding racing venues.

7. Challenges and Resilience in Economic Models:

- Navigating Financial Challenges: The industry faces various financial challenges, including fluctuations in betting revenue, increased competition from other forms of entertainment, and public scrutiny. This section explores how the greyhound racing community navigates these challenges and adapts its economic models to ensure resilience.

- Innovations in Revenue Generation: To sustain and grow, the industry explores innovative ways to diversify its revenue streams. The chapter discusses how advancements in technology, partnerships, and fan engagement initiatives contribute to the ongoing evolution of the industry's economic models.

Conclusion - Balancing Act of Economics and Passion:

The economic dynamics of greyhound racing represent a delicate balance between financial sustainability and the passion that drives the sport. As the industry navigates the complexities of revenue generation and operational costs, it continually adapts to ensure that the economic underpinnings support the well-being of greyhounds, the livelihoods of those involved, and the enduring appeal of this exhilarating sport.

Media Deals and Broadcasting

In the modern era, the success and visibility of greyhound racing are intricately tied to media deals and broadcasting arrangements. This chapter explores the symbiotic relationship between the racing industry and the media, examining how partnerships, technological advancements, and the dissemination of content contribute to the sport's widespread appeal and economic viability.

1. Evolution of Media Coverage:

- From Local Tracks to Global Screens: The chapter opens by tracing the evolution of media coverage in greyhound racing. It explores how the sport transitioned from local track events to gaining a global audience through various media channels, including television, radio, and, more recently, online streaming platforms.

- Impact of Technological Advancements: Technological advancements have revolutionized the way greyhound racing is presented and consumed. This section delves into the impact of innovations such as high-definition broadcasts, slow-motion replays, and virtual reality experiences on the viewing experience and fan engagement.

2. Television Broadcasting:

- Strategic Partnerships with Networks: Television broadcasting remains a cornerstone of the sport's media presence. The chapter examines how greyhound racing organizations strategically partner with television networks to secure coverage, ensuring that races reach a broad and diverse audience.

- Production Quality and Commentary: The quality of production and the expertise of commentators significantly influence the viewer experience. This section explores how racing organizations invest in production value, camera angles, and insightful commentary to enhance the overall appeal of televised greyhound racing.

3. Online Streaming Platforms:

- The Rise of Online Streaming: The advent of online streaming platforms has democratized access to greyhound racing content. This part of the chapter discusses how racing organizations leverage streaming services to reach a global audience, offering live broadcasts, race archives, and exclusive behind-the-scenes content.

- Interactive Fan Engagement: Online platforms provide opportunities for interactive fan engagement. This section explores how live chats, social media integration, and virtual fan experiences enhance viewer participation, fostering a sense of community among greyhound racing enthusiasts.

4. Radio Broadcasting and Podcasts:

- Capturing the Thrill through Audio: While visuals are integral, audio broadcasts hold a unique place in capturing the excitement of greyhound racing. The chapter explores the role of radio broadcasting in conveying the thrill of races, and how podcasts contribute to in-depth discussions, interviews, and analysis.

- Accessibility and Inclusivity: Radio and podcasts enhance the accessibility and inclusivity of greyhound racing content. This section discusses how these audio formats cater to a diverse audience, including those who prefer on-the-go listening and those who may have visual impairments.

5. Sponsorship Integration and Commercial Partnerships:

- Branding Opportunities for Sponsors: Media deals offer valuable branding opportunities for sponsors. This part of the chapter examines how sponsors and commercial partners integrate their branding into broadcasts, from race sponsorships to logo placements and promotional segments.

- Mutually Beneficial Partnerships: Successful media deals are built on mutually beneficial partnerships between racing organizations and sponsors. The section explores how these collaborations go beyond traditional advertising, creating engaging and authentic connections with the audience.

6. Challenges and Innovations in Media Deals:

- Navigating Challenges in Traditional Media: The chapter discusses challenges faced by greyhound racing in traditional media, including competition for airtime, changing viewer habits, and negotiating broadcasting rights. It explores how the industry navigates these challenges and adapts its strategies.

- Innovations in Digital Media: Digital media presents both opportunities and challenges. This section examines how the racing industry innovates in the digital space, from exclusive online streaming deals to partnerships with emerging platforms, ensuring that the sport remains at the forefront of digital engagement.

7. International Broadcasting and Global Appeal:

- Showcasing the Sport to a Global Audience: Greyhound racing's global appeal is amplified through international broadcasting. This part of the chapter explores how the sport reaches audiences in different countries, showcasing the diversity of tracks, events, and racing cultures.

- Cultural Sensitivity and Adaptation: Broadcasting internationally requires a nuanced approach to cultural sensitivity and adaptation. The chapter discusses how the racing industry tailors its content and commentary to resonate with diverse audiences while respecting local sensitivities.

Conclusion - The Future of Greyhound Racing on Screens:

The concluding section reflects on the ever-evolving landscape of media deals and broadcasting in greyhound racing. It explores how the industry anticipates and adapts to future technological advancements, changing viewer preferences, and emerging media platforms, ensuring that the sport continues to captivate audiences around the world through innovative and engaging content.

Gambling and Bookmaking

Greyhound racing has long been synonymous with the thrill of wagering, making gambling and bookmaking integral components of the sport's economic landscape. This chapter explores the intricate world of betting on greyhound races, the role of bookmakers, and the symbiotic relationship between the racing industry and the gambling economy.

1. Historical Roots of Betting:

- Early Wagering Practices: The chapter begins by delving into the historical roots of betting on greyhound races. From informal wagers among spectators to the emergence of organized betting at racetracks, it traces how gambling became inextricably linked with the sport.

- The Evolution of Betting Culture: Over the years, the betting culture around greyhound racing has evolved. This section explores the shift from informal, localized betting to the establishment of formalized systems, laying the groundwork for the sophisticated gambling practices seen in the contemporary era.

2. Types of Bets and Betting Strategies:

- Straight Bets and Exotic Wagers: The chapter provides an in-depth exploration of the various types of bets available to greyhound racing enthusiasts. From straightforward win, place, and show bets to exotic wagers like trifectas and exactas, it details the diverse range of betting options.

- Betting Strategies and Systems: Racing enthusiasts often employ different strategies and systems to inform their betting decisions. This section delves into popular betting strategies, including form analysis, handicapping, and statistical approaches that punters use to gain an edge.

3. The Role of Bookmakers:

- Bookmaking Operations: Bookmakers play a central role in facilitating betting on greyhound races. The chapter explores how bookmaking operations function, from setting odds to managing risk, and highlights the responsibilities of bookmakers in ensuring fair and transparent betting environments.

- Online Bookmakers and Technological Advancements: The advent of online bookmaking platforms has transformed the industry. This section examines how technological advancements have enabled the rise of online bookmakers, expanding the accessibility and convenience of betting for enthusiasts around the world.

4. Wagering Platforms and Technology:

- On-Site Betting Facilities: Traditional on-site betting facilities at racetracks remain popular among spectators. The chapter discusses how these facilities operate, providing insights into the atmosphere, services, and technologies that enhance the on-site betting experience.

- Online Betting Platforms and Mobile Apps: The convenience of online betting platforms and mobile apps has revolutionized the industry. This part of the chapter explores the proliferation of online bookmakers, mobile betting apps, and the role of technology in shaping the contemporary landscape of greyhound racing gambling.

5. Responsible Gambling Practices:

- Promoting Responsible Betting: The chapter emphasizes the importance of promoting responsible gambling practices within the greyhound racing community. It explores initiatives undertaken by the industry to address issues related to problem gambling and ensure the well-being of participants and spectators.

- Education and Support Programs: Racing organizations actively engage in educational and support programs to foster responsible gambling. This section delves into the various initiatives, such as awareness campaigns, counseling services, and self-exclusion programs, aimed at mitigating the potential harms associated with excessive gambling.

6. Gambling and Revenue Generation:

- Economic Significance of Gambling: Gambling is a key driver of revenue for the greyhound racing industry. This part of the chapter explores the economic significance of betting, examining how the proceeds from gambling contribute to prize pools, track maintenance, and overall financial sustainability.

- Impact on Racing Dynamics: Beyond its economic role, gambling also influences the dynamics of greyhound racing. This section discusses how the presence of betting enhances the competitive nature of races, attracting top-tier competitors and fostering a vibrant and engaging racing environment.

7. Challenges and Regulatory Framework:

- Regulating the Gambling Ecosystem: The chapter addresses the regulatory framework that governs greyhound racing gambling. It explores the challenges associated with ensuring fairness, preventing fraudulent activities, and maintaining the integrity of betting in a rapidly evolving technological landscape.

- Addressing Ethical Concerns: Ethical considerations, such as the welfare of racing greyhounds and the potential for exploitation, are critical aspects of the gambling ecosystem. This section examines how the industry addresses these concerns through ethical guidelines, transparency, and stakeholder engagement.

Conclusion - Balancing the Thrill with Responsibility:

In conclusion, the chapter reflects on the delicate balance between the thrill of gambling and the responsibility to ensure a fair, transparent, and ethical betting environment within the greyhound racing industry. It underscores the ongoing efforts to preserve the excitement of wagering while prioritizing the welfare of participants and the integrity of the sport.

Regulation and State Oversight

Greyhound racing, like any organized sport involving competition and wagering, is subject to comprehensive regulation and state oversight. This chapter examines the intricate web of rules, agencies, and ethical considerations that shape the industry, ensuring the fair conduct of races, the well-being of greyhounds, and the integrity of the entire enterprise.

1. Historical Evolution of Regulation:

- Early Attempts at Oversight: The chapter opens by exploring the historical evolution of regulation in greyhound racing. It delves into the early attempts at oversight, examining how rudimentary rules gradually evolved into a sophisticated regulatory framework in response to the growth and commercialization of the sport.

- Regulatory Milestones: Highlighting key milestones, this section discusses significant moments in the establishment and refinement of regulations governing greyhound racing. It explores how these milestones reflect the industry's commitment to enhancing transparency, fairness, and ethical standards.

2. Agencies and Authorities:

- State Racing Commissions: State racing commissions play a pivotal role in overseeing greyhound racing within their jurisdictions. The chapter examines the functions and responsibilities of these commissions, including licensing, rule enforcement, and the adjudication of disputes to maintain the integrity of the sport.

- Role of National Organizations: National organizations, such as the National Greyhound Association

(NGA), also contribute to the regulatory landscape. This section explores their role in setting standards, facilitating communication among stakeholders, and promoting uniformity in regulations across different states.

3. Licensing and Compliance:

- Owner, Trainer, and Handler Licensing: Licensing is a crucial aspect of regulation, ensuring that individuals involved in greyhound racing meet specified standards. This part of the chapter delves into the licensing requirements for owners, trainers, handlers, and other key personnel, emphasizing the need for competence and ethical conduct.

- Kennel and Track Compliance: Beyond individual licensing, the regulation extends to kennels and racetracks. This section explores how regulatory bodies enforce compliance standards for kennel facilities and tracks, covering aspects such as animal welfare, track maintenance, and safety protocols.

4. Integrity and Anti-Corruption Measures:

- Ensuring Fair Play: Maintaining the integrity of greyhound racing is paramount. The chapter discusses the measures in place to prevent cheating, race-fixing, and other forms of corruption. It explores how surveillance, investigation, and penalties contribute to a level playing field for all participants.

- Anti-Doping Protocols: Greyhound racing incorporates anti-doping measures to ensure that competing dogs are not subjected to performance-enhancing substances. This section details the protocols in place, including drug testing procedures and the consequences for violations.

5. Animal Welfare Regulations:

- Health and Safety Standards: The welfare of racing greyhounds is a central focus of regulation. This part of the chapter delves into the health and safety standards that govern the treatment of greyhounds, addressing issues such as housing conditions, veterinary care, and humane euthanasia practices.

- Retirement and Adoption Protocols: Regulations also guide the retirement and adoption processes for racing greyhounds. This section explores how the industry ensures that retired dogs transition to post-racing life with care, emphasizing adoption programs and partnerships with rescue organizations.

6. Public Perception and Ethical Considerations:

- Community Engagement: The chapter discusses how regulatory bodies engage with the public and stakeholders to address concerns, promote transparency, and build trust. It explores initiatives that foster communication, education, and collaboration between regulators, industry participants, and the broader community.

- Ethical Considerations in Regulation: Ethical considerations are inherent in greyhound racing regulation. This section examines how regulations evolve to reflect changing societal norms, with a focus on ethical treatment of animals, responsible gambling practices, and fair competition.

7. Evolving Regulatory Challenges:

- Adapting to Technological Changes: Regulatory challenges evolve alongside technological advancements. This section explores how the industry navigates challenges posed by emerging technologies, online betting platforms, and the need for updated surveillance and enforcement mechanisms.

- Addressing Public Concerns: Public perception and concerns can influence regulatory priorities. The chapter discusses how regulatory bodies proactively address public concerns, incorporating feedback, and implementing changes that align with evolving expectations regarding animal welfare, safety, and fairness.

Conclusion - Nurturing a Responsible Industry:

In conclusion, the chapter reflects on the dynamic nature of greyhound racing regulation and state oversight. It emphasizes the industry's commitment to continuous improvement, transparency, and ethical practices to ensure that the sport thrives responsibly, maintaining the delicate balance between competition, entertainment, and the welfare of all participants.

Challenges from Animal Rights Groups

Greyhound racing, like many animal-centric sports, faces significant scrutiny and challenges from animal rights groups. This chapter explores the concerns raised by these groups, the evolving landscape of public opinion, and the industry's responses to ensure the welfare of racing greyhounds.

1. Origins of Animal Rights Advocacy:

- Emergence of Animal Rights Movements: The chapter begins by tracing the roots of animal rights advocacy and its evolution into a prominent social movement. It explores how concerns for the welfare of animals, including those involved in sports like greyhound racing, gained momentum over time.

- Focus on Greyhound Racing: As part of the broader animal rights discourse, this section delves into why greyhound racing has become a focal point for advocacy. It examines factors such as the perception of exploitation, concerns about breeding practices, and incidents that have fueled public outcry.

2. Welfare Concerns and Criticisms:

- Issues of Exploitation and Mistreatment: Animal rights groups often raise concerns about the perceived exploitation and mistreatment of racing greyhounds. This part of the chapter examines specific instances that have triggered controversies, shedding light on practices that activists find objectionable.

- Challenges to Racing Practices: The chapter explores criticisms directed at various aspects of greyhound racing, including the use of mechanical lures, confinement conditions in kennels, and the physical demands placed on racing dogs. It delves into how these concerns have prompted calls for reform within the industry.

3. High-Profile Cases and Investigations:

- Impact of Exposés and Investigations: High-profile cases and investigations have played a pivotal role in shaping public perception. This section explores the impact of exposés and investigations on greyhound racing, examining how media coverage has influenced public sentiment and intensified scrutiny.

- Industry Responses to Allegations: To provide a comprehensive view, the chapter discusses how the greyhound racing industry has responded to allegations raised by animal rights groups. It examines proactive measures, changes in regulations, and collaborative efforts to address concerns and improve practices.

4. Legislative and Regulatory Reforms:

- Changing Legal Landscape: The legal framework surrounding greyhound racing has experienced shifts in response to animal rights advocacy. This part of the chapter examines legislative changes aimed at enhancing the welfare of racing greyhounds, including bans on certain practices and increased oversight.

- Regulatory Adaptations: Regulatory bodies have adapted to changing expectations and concerns. This section explores how racing commissions and national organizations have revised regulations, implemented new standards, and collaborated with stakeholders to align the industry with evolving ethical standards.

5. Industry-Driven Welfare Initiatives:

- Retirement and Adoption Programs: Recognizing the need for post-racing care, the industry has initiated retirement and adoption programs for greyhounds. The chapter explores these programs, highlighting collaborations with rescue organizations and efforts to ensure that retired dogs find loving homes.

- Investments in Canine Welfare: Industry stakeholders have made investments in veterinary care, housing conditions, and overall canine welfare. This section details these initiatives, emphasizing the commitment to enhancing the well-being of racing greyhounds both during their careers and in retirement.

6. Collaboration with Advocacy Groups:

- Engaging with Animal Rights Organizations: The chapter discusses instances of collaboration between the greyhound racing industry and animal rights organizations. It explores how dialogue and partnership initiatives aim to find common ground, address concerns, and foster a more transparent and accountable industry.

- Impact of Collaboration on Industry Practices: Examining the outcomes of collaboration, this section assesses how partnerships with advocacy groups have influenced industry practices, from improved transparency and accountability to joint initiatives promoting the welfare of racing greyhounds.

7. Public Awareness and Education:

- Communication Strategies: Recognizing the importance of public perception, the industry has engaged in communication strategies to raise awareness about its commitment to animal welfare. This part of the chapter explores how these efforts aim to convey a more balanced and accurate portrayal of greyhound racing.

- Educational Programs: Educational programs targeting the public, racing enthusiasts, and industry participants play a role in dispelling misconceptions. The chapter discusses initiatives that provide insights into the care, training, and retirement of racing greyhounds to foster a better-informed public.

Conclusion - Navigating a Complex Landscape:

In conclusion, the chapter reflects on the complex landscape of challenges presented by animal rights groups to the greyhound racing industry. It emphasizes the ongoing efforts to address concerns, implement reforms, and collaborate with stakeholders to ensure the welfare of racing greyhounds while acknowledging the importance of maintaining a sustainable and ethical sporting environment.

Chapter 9: Greyhound Racing by Region
The Sport's Roots in Florida and the South

Greyhound racing's journey in the United States is intrinsically tied to the South, particularly the state of Florida, where its roots run deep. This section delves into the historical context, the development of racing culture, and the pivotal role played by Florida and the Southern states in shaping the landscape of greyhound racing.

1. Early Days of Greyhound Racing in Florida:

- Introduction to Greyhound Racing in Florida: The chapter begins by setting the stage for the emergence of greyhound racing in Florida. It explores how the state became a focal point for the sport, driven by a combination of favorable climate, economic factors, and the Southern tradition of dog racing.

- Pioneering Tracks and Events: Delving into the early tracks and events, this section traces the pioneers who laid the foundation for greyhound racing in Florida. It discusses the inaugural races, the enthusiasm of spectators, and the gradual evolution of the sport within the region.

2. Florida's Role in Shaping Racing Culture:

- Cultural Impact of Greyhound Racing: Greyhound racing became more than just a sport; it embedded itself in the cultural fabric of Florida. This part of the chapter examines how the sport influenced the local culture, from social activities to the development of a unique racing community.

- Racing as Entertainment: Greyhound racing in Florida transcended being solely a competitive event. It became a form of entertainment, drawing crowds not only for the thrill of the races but also for the social experience and the sense of community fostered at the tracks.

3. Expansion Across the Southern States:

- Spread to Surrounding States: The chapter explores the natural expansion of greyhound racing from Florida to neighboring Southern states. It discusses how the sport gained popularity across the region, with new tracks emerging and contributing to the growth of the industry.

- Southern Racing Culture: Greyhound racing took on a distinct Southern flavor as it expanded. This section delves into the unique aspects of racing culture in the Southern states, examining traditions, events, and the role of greyhound racing in the broader Southern lifestyle.

4. Economic Impact on the Region:

- Job Creation and Economic Stimulus: Greyhound racing brought about economic benefits to the region, creating jobs and stimulating local economies. This part of the chapter examines the economic impact, from the employment opportunities provided by racing facilities to the influx of visitors and revenue.

- Tourism and Hospitality: The sport became a draw for tourists, further contributing to the economic landscape. The chapter explores how greyhound racing in the South became intertwined with the tourism and hospitality sectors, attracting visitors and bolstering the region's appeal.

5. Notable Tracks and Events in Florida and the South:

- Iconic Tracks: Highlighting key tracks in Florida and the Southern states, this section explores the iconic venues that became synonymous with greyhound racing. It discusses their significance, architecture, and contributions to the overall racing experience.

- Signature Events: The chapter delves into signature events hosted in the region, showcasing races that became annual highlights. It explores the traditions, rituals, and unique features that distinguished these events and attracted racing enthusiasts.

6. Challenges and Transformations:

- Impact of Changing Dynamics: The chapter acknowledges the challenges faced by greyhound racing in Florida and the South. It discusses how changing societal attitudes, economic shifts, and regulatory developments have influenced the sport's trajectory in the region.

- Adaptations and Transformations: Examining the responses to challenges, this section discusses how the industry has adapted and transformed. It explores initiatives aimed at modernizing the sport, enhancing its appeal, and addressing concerns to secure its future in the Southern states.

Conclusion - Legacy and Evolution:

In conclusion, the chapter reflects on the enduring legacy of greyhound racing in Florida and the Southern states. It acknowledges the sport's historical significance, cultural impact, and economic contributions while recognizing the need for continued adaptation to navigate the evolving landscape of the industry in this region.

Tracks and Styles Across the Western US

The Western United States has its own rich tapestry of greyhound racing, with distinctive tracks, racing styles, and a unique racing culture. This section explores the evolution of greyhound racing in the Western US, highlighting key tracks, regional variations, and the contributions of the Western states to the broader landscape of the sport.

1. Early Development of Greyhound Racing in the West:

- Introduction to Western US Racing: The chapter opens with an exploration of how greyhound racing found its way to the Western United States. It discusses the initial tracks, the reception from local communities, and the factors that contributed to the sport's establishment in the region.

- Influence of Western Culture: Examining the influence of Western culture on greyhound racing, this section delves into how the sport adapted to and integrated with the unique characteristics of the Western US. It explores the symbiotic relationship between the sport and the region's cultural identity.

2. Key Tracks and Racing Hubs:

- Prominent Western Tracks: Highlighting key tracks in the Western US, this part of the chapter discusses the prominent venues that became integral to the regional racing scene. It explores the architecture, historical significance, and contributions of these tracks to the Western greyhound racing landscape.

- Racing Hubs and Clusters: Examining the clustering of tracks in certain regions, the chapter delves into how racing hubs developed and contributed to the overall vibrancy of greyhound racing in the Western states. It discusses the interplay between tracks, competition, and collaboration.

3. Regional Variations in Racing Styles:

- Distinctive Western Racing Styles: Greyhound racing in the Western US developed its own distinctive styles and characteristics. This section explores how factors such as track configurations, weather conditions, and local preferences influenced the evolution of racing styles in the region.

- Influence of Terrain and Climate: The chapter delves into how the varied terrain and climate of the Western states impacted racing styles. From desert tracks to those nestled in mountainous regions, it examines how environmental factors shaped the way races were conducted.

4. Integration with Western Sporting Culture:

- Greyhound Racing as a Western Sport: Greyhound racing became more than an event; it became part of the sporting culture in the Western US. This part of the chapter explores how the sport integrated with existing Western sports culture, drawing parallels with rodeos, horse racing, and other regional sporting traditions.

- Local Racing Traditions: Examining local racing traditions, the chapter discusses how specific regions within the Western US developed their own rituals, celebrations, and events around greyhound racing. It explores how these traditions added depth to the overall racing experience.

5. Economic Impact and Tourism:

- Economic Contributions: Greyhound racing made substantial economic contributions to the Western states. This section examines the job creation, revenue generation, and economic impact of the sport on local communities, emphasizing its role in supporting livelihoods and businesses.

- Tourism and Spectatorship: The chapter explores how greyhound racing in the Western US attracted visitors and contributed to tourism. It discusses the allure of regional racing events, the influx of spectators, and the symbiotic relationship between the sport and the hospitality industry.

6. Challenges and Innovations:

- Challenges Faced by Western Tracks: Acknowledging the challenges faced by greyhound racing in the Western US, this section discusses the impact of changing demographics, regulatory shifts, and other factors. It explores how tracks navigated challenges and adapted to ensure their continued viability.

- Innovations in Western Greyhound Racing: Examining innovations in response to challenges, the chapter discusses how Western tracks embraced new technologies, marketing strategies, and racing formats. It explores initiatives aimed at modernizing the sport while preserving its cultural and regional identity.

Conclusion - Western Greyhound Racing Legacy:

In conclusion, the chapter reflects on the enduring legacy of greyhound racing in the Western United States. It recognizes the unique contributions of the region to the broader tapestry of the sport, celebrating the rich history, cultural integration, and ongoing adaptations that define Western greyhound racing.

Midwestern Racing Heritage and Culture

The Midwest holds a significant place in the history and culture of greyhound racing in the United States. This section explores the development of greyhound racing in the Midwest, tracing its roots, examining key tracks, and delving into the unique racing culture that has flourished in this region.

1. Early Development and Pioneering Tracks:

- Emergence of Greyhound Racing in the Midwest: The chapter begins by exploring how greyhound racing found its way to the Midwest and became an integral part of the region's sporting landscape. It discusses the factors that contributed to the sport's early development in Midwestern states.

- Pioneering Tracks and Influential Figures: Delving into the history of the first tracks in the Midwest, this section highlights the pioneers and influential individuals who played a key role in establishing greyhound racing in the region. It examines their contributions to the growth of the sport.

2. Cultural Integration and Midwestern Traditions:

- Cultural Significance of Greyhound Racing: Greyhound racing became intertwined with Midwestern culture, influencing social traditions and becoming a staple in the region's sporting calendar. This part of the chapter explores how the sport integrated with the cultural fabric of the Midwest.

- Local Racing Traditions: Examining regional racing traditions, the chapter discusses how specific Midwestern states developed their own rituals, celebrations, and events around greyhound racing. It explores the unique traditions that emerged and contributed to the overall racing experience.

3. Iconic Tracks and Racing Hubs:

- Prominent Midwestern Tracks: Highlighting key tracks in the Midwest, this section discusses the iconic venues that became central to the regional racing scene. It explores the architecture, historical significance, and contributions of these tracks to the Midwestern greyhound racing landscape.

- Racing Hubs and Clusters: Examining the clustering of tracks in certain regions, the chapter delves into how racing hubs developed in the Midwest. It discusses the interplay between tracks, competition, and collaboration, contributing to the vibrancy of greyhound racing in the region.

4. Racing Styles and Variations:

- Distinctive Midwestern Racing Styles: Greyhound racing in the Midwest developed its own distinctive styles and characteristics. This section explores how factors such as track configurations, weather conditions, and local preferences influenced the evolution of racing styles in the region.

- Impact of Topography and Climate: The chapter delves into how the Midwestern topography and climate impacted racing styles. From flat tracks to those with slight inclines, it examines how environmental factors shaped the way races were conducted in the region.

5. Economic Contributions and Community Impact:

- Economic Contributions: Greyhound racing made substantial economic contributions to the Midwest. This section examines the job creation, revenue generation, and economic impact of the sport on local communities, emphasizing its role in supporting livelihoods and businesses.

- Community Engagement and Support: The chapter explores the community engagement fostered by greyhound racing in the Midwest. It discusses how the sport became a rallying point, bringing people together and fostering a sense of local pride and identity.

6. Challenges and Resilience:

- Challenges Faced by Midwestern Tracks: Acknowledging the challenges faced by greyhound racing in the Midwest, this section discusses the impact of changing demographics, regulatory shifts, and other factors. It explores how tracks navigated challenges and adapted to ensure their continued viability.

- Resilience and Adaptation: Examining resilience in the face of challenges, the chapter discusses how Midwestern tracks embraced new technologies, marketing strategies, and racing formats. It explores initiatives aimed at modernizing the sport while preserving its cultural and regional identity.

Conclusion - Midwestern Greyhound Racing Legacy:

In conclusion, the chapter reflects on the enduring legacy of greyhound racing in the Midwest. It recognizes the unique contributions of the region to the broader tapestry of the sport, celebrating the rich history, cultural integration, and ongoing adaptations that define Midwestern greyhound racing.

New England's Connections to Greyhound Racing

New England, known for its rich history and distinct culture, has played a unique role in the development of greyhound racing in the United States. This section explores the connections between New England and greyhound racing, tracing the sport's roots in the region, examining key tracks, and delving into the cultural impact of greyhound racing on New England.

1. Early Greyhound Racing in New England:

- Introduction to Greyhound Racing in New England: The chapter begins by providing an overview of how greyhound racing became a part of New England's sporting landscape. It discusses the early days of the sport in the region, examining the factors that contributed to its establishment.

- Pioneering Tracks and Influential Figures: Delving into the history of the first greyhound racing tracks in New England, this section highlights the pioneers and influential individuals who played a key role in establishing the sport in the region. It explores their contributions to the growth of greyhound racing.

2. Cultural Integration and New England Traditions:

- Cultural Significance of Greyhound Racing in New England: Greyhound racing became more than a sport; it became a cultural phenomenon in New England. This part of the chapter explores how the sport integrated with the cultural fabric of the region, influencing traditions and social activities.

- Local Racing Traditions: Examining regional racing traditions, the chapter discusses how specific states in New England developed their own rituals, celebrations, and events around greyhound racing. It explores the unique traditions that emerged and contributed to the overall racing experience.

3. Iconic Tracks and Racing Hubs:

- Prominent New England Tracks: Highlighting key tracks in New England, this section discusses the iconic venues that became central to the regional racing scene. It explores the architecture, historical significance, and contributions of these tracks to the New England greyhound racing landscape.

- Racing Hubs and Community Engagement: Examining the clustering of tracks in certain regions, the chapter delves into how racing hubs developed in New England. It discusses the interplay between tracks, competition, and community engagement, contributing to the vibrancy of greyhound racing in the region.

4. Racing Styles and Environmental Influences:

- Distinctive New England Racing Styles: Greyhound racing in New England developed its own distinctive styles and characteristics. This section explores how factors such as track configurations, weather conditions, and local preferences influenced the evolution of racing styles in the region.

- Impact of Geography and Climate: The chapter delves into how the geography and climate of New England impacted racing styles. From coastal tracks to those nestled in hilly landscapes, it examines how environmental factors shaped the way races were conducted.

5. Economic Contributions and Local Impact:

- Economic Contributions: Greyhound racing made substantial economic contributions to New England. This section examines the job creation, revenue generation, and economic impact of the sport on local communities, emphasizing its role in supporting livelihoods and businesses.

- Community Engagement and Social Impact: The chapter explores how greyhound racing in New England fostered community engagement. It discusses the social impact of the sport, its role in bringing people together, and the sense of identity and pride it instilled in local communities.

6. Challenges and Adaptations:

- Challenges Faced by New England Tracks: Acknowledging the challenges faced by greyhound racing in New England, this section discusses the impact of changing demographics, regulatory shifts, and other factors. It explores how tracks navigated challenges and adapted to ensure their continued viability.

- Innovations and Preservation Efforts: Examining innovations in response to challenges, the chapter discusses how New England tracks embraced new technologies, marketing strategies, and racing formats. It explores initiatives aimed at modernizing the sport while preserving its cultural and regional identity.

Conclusion - New England Greyhound Racing Legacy:

In conclusion, the chapter reflects on the enduring legacy of greyhound racing in New England. It recognizes the unique contributions of the region to the broader tapestry of the sport, celebrating the rich history, cultural integration, and ongoing adaptations that define New England's connection to greyhound racing.

Greyhound racing has transcended national borders, becoming a global phenomenon with strong roots in the United Kingdom, Ireland, and Australia. This section explores the history, culture, and unique characteristics of greyhound racing in these international hubs, highlighting the role each region has played in shaping the sport on a global scale.

1. United Kingdom: Pioneering the Modern Era

- Historical Evolution: The chapter begins by tracing the historical evolution of greyhound racing in the United Kingdom. From its humble beginnings to the establishment of the first tracks, it explores how the sport gained popularity and became an integral part of British culture.

- The Modern Racing Scene: Examining the contemporary landscape, this section delves into the modern era of greyhound racing in the UK. It discusses the key tracks, major events, and the evolution of the sport, highlighting how it has adapted to changing times.

- Cultural Significance: Greyhound racing in the UK goes beyond sport; it is deeply embedded in the culture. This part of the chapter explores the cultural significance of greyhound racing, including traditions, social aspects, and its portrayal in the media.

2. Ireland: The Emerald Isle's Racing Heritage

- Introduction to Irish Greyhound Racing: The focus shifts to Ireland, exploring how greyhound racing became a cherished pastime on the Emerald Isle. It delves into the historical factors that contributed to the sport's establishment and growth in Ireland.

- Prominent Irish Tracks and Events: Highlighting key tracks and events, this section discusses the racing hubs that have become iconic in Ireland. It explores the unique characteristics of Irish greyhound racing and the major competitions that draw enthusiasts from around the world.

- Cross-Cultural Influences: Examining the cross-cultural influences between Ireland and other greyhound racing nations, the chapter discusses how Irish breeding, racing styles, and expertise have contributed to the global development of the sport.

3. Australia: A Sporting Nation's Passion

- Greyhound Racing Down Under: Shifting focus to Australia, the chapter explores the roots of greyhound racing in the country. It discusses the early days, the establishment of tracks, and the factors that led to the sport's widespread popularity among Australians.

- Notable Australian Tracks and Competitions: Highlighting significant tracks and competitions, this section delves into the diverse racing landscape in Australia. It discusses the unique characteristics of Australian greyhound racing and profiles major events that capture the nation's attention.

- Impact on Australian Culture: Greyhound racing has become ingrained in Australian culture. This part of the chapter explores how the sport has influenced the national identity, traditions associated with racing, and its representation in Australian popular culture.

4. Global Collaboration and Competition:

- International Competitions and Exchange: Greyhound racing in the UK, Ireland, and Australia has fostered international collaboration. This section explores how these nations participate in global competitions, exchange breeding expertise, and contribute to the overall growth of the sport.

- Challenges and Opportunities in International Racing: Discussing the challenges faced by international greyhound racing, the chapter explores regulatory differences, ethical considerations, and the opportunities for collaboration to address common issues. It considers how these regions navigate the complexities of a globalized racing landscape.

5. Future Trends and Innovations:

- Technological Advancements: The chapter looks ahead to the future of greyhound racing in these international hubs, exploring how technological advancements are shaping the sport. It discusses innovations in track infrastructure, race analysis, and fan engagement.

- Sustainability and Welfare: Examining the growing emphasis on sustainability and greyhound welfare, this section discusses how these regions are adapting to meet evolving societal expectations and addressing concerns related to the treatment of racing greyhounds.

Conclusion - Global Legacy of Greyhound Racing:

In conclusion, the chapter reflects on the global legacy of greyhound racing rooted in the UK, Ireland, and Australia. It acknowledges the impact of each region on the sport's development, celebrating the cultural richness, racing traditions, and ongoing contributions to the international greyhound racing community.

Chapter 10: The Future of Greyhound Racing
Changing Public Perceptions and Ethical Concerns

Greyhound racing faces a pivotal juncture as shifting societal attitudes and heightened ethical concerns prompt a reevaluation of the sport. This section explores the evolving public perceptions surrounding greyhound racing and the ethical considerations that are reshaping its landscape.

1. Historical Context of Public Perceptions:

- Early Positive Reception: The chapter begins by examining the historical context of public perceptions toward greyhound racing. Initially celebrated for its excitement and athleticism, the sport enjoyed positive reception, contributing to its widespread popularity.

- Shifts in Public Opinion: Over time, public sentiments have shifted, influenced by evolving societal values, increased awareness of animal welfare, and changes in ethical standards. This section explores the factors that have contributed to the changing narrative surrounding greyhound racing.

2. Animal Welfare and Ethical Concerns:

- Injuries and Health Issues: A critical aspect of changing perceptions revolves around the welfare of racing greyhounds. The chapter delves into the ethical concerns raised by injuries and health issues suffered by racing dogs, examining the impact on both individual animals and the sport as a whole.

- Scientific Studies on Breed Welfare: Building on the earlier discussion, this section explores scientific studies that have investigated the welfare of greyhounds in racing. It discusses research findings, highlighting areas of concern and potential areas for improvement.

- Doping Scandals and Prevention Efforts: The chapter examines the ethical implications of doping scandals within the greyhound racing industry. It explores efforts to prevent doping, the impact on the health and fair competition of greyhounds, and the broader implications for the sport.

3. Ethics of Breeding Practices and Culling:

- Selective Breeding Practices: This section addresses the ethical considerations surrounding selective breeding in greyhound racing. It discusses the pursuit of specific traits and the potential implications for the overall health and well-being of the breed.

- Culling Practices: The chapter explores the controversial practice of culling, examining instances where dogs deemed unsuitable for racing are culled. It delves into the ethical dimensions of culling and alternative approaches aimed at ensuring the welfare of retired or non-competitive greyhounds.

4. Retirement and Adoption Initiatives:

- Retirement Programs: Recognizing the importance of responsible aftercare, the chapter discusses retirement programs implemented within the greyhound racing community. It explores efforts to transition racing dogs into post-racing life, emphasizing the responsibility of owners and the industry.

- Adoption Efforts and Success Stories: This section highlights adoption initiatives that aim to provide retired greyhounds with loving homes. It shares success stories of greyhounds thriving in their post-racing lives, showcasing positive outcomes resulting from adoption efforts.

5. Industry Responses to Ethical Concerns:

- Regulatory Reforms: The chapter examines how the greyhound racing industry is responding to ethical concerns through regulatory reforms. It discusses changes in rules and standards aimed at enhancing the welfare of racing dogs.

- Transparency and Accountability: This section explores the role of transparency and accountability in addressing ethical concerns. It discusses initiatives within the industry to improve transparency regarding the treatment of greyhounds, racing conditions, and breeding practices.

6. Public Awareness and Advocacy:

- Impact of Public Awareness: Public awareness campaigns have played a crucial role in shaping perceptions of greyhound racing. The chapter explores the impact of these campaigns in influencing public opinion, fostering awareness of ethical concerns, and driving change.

- Role of Animal Rights Groups: Examining the role of animal rights groups, the section discusses how advocacy organizations have contributed to raising ethical standards within the greyhound racing industry. It explores collaborative efforts between stakeholders and advocacy groups.

7. Balancing Tradition with Ethical Progress:

- Preserving Racing Traditions: Acknowledging the deep-seated traditions within greyhound racing, this part of the chapter discusses the challenges of balancing tradition with evolving ethical considerations. It explores how the sport can adapt without losing its historical and cultural significance.

- Innovations for Ethical Racing: Looking toward the future, the chapter explores innovations that can enhance the ethical aspects of greyhound racing. It discusses technological advancements, policy changes, and industry-wide initiatives aimed at fostering a more ethical and sustainable sport.

Conclusion - Navigating the Path Forward:

In conclusion, the chapter reflects on the dynamic interplay between changing public perceptions and ethical considerations in the world of greyhound racing. It considers the ongoing efforts to address concerns, foster responsible practices, and navigate the path forward, ensuring the sport's viability while upholding ethical standards.

Shifting Legislative Landscape and Regulations

As greyhound racing grapples with evolving societal expectations and ethical concerns, the legislative landscape and regulatory framework become central to shaping the future of the sport. This section explores the dynamic interplay between the shifting legislative landscape and the regulations governing greyhound racing.

1. Historical Overview of Legislation:

- Early Regulation and Oversight: The chapter begins by providing a historical overview of legislation related to greyhound racing. It explores the early stages of regulation and oversight, examining the formation of rules to ensure fair competition and the welfare of racing greyhounds.

- Legislative Milestones: Tracing legislative milestones, this section highlights key moments in the history of greyhound racing regulations. It discusses how regulations have adapted to address emerging challenges and societal expectations over the years.

2. Contemporary Legislative Developments:

- Recent Reforms and Changes: The chapter shifts focus to contemporary legislative developments. It examines recent reforms and changes in regulations aimed at addressing ethical concerns, improving transparency, and safeguarding the welfare of racing greyhounds.

- Public-Private Collaboration: Highlighting the collaborative efforts between government bodies and private entities, this section discusses how the legislative landscape has evolved to accommodate input from various stakeholders, including industry experts, animal welfare advocates, and the public.

3. Ethical Imperatives Driving Legislation:

- Public Sentiment and Advocacy Impact: The chapter explores how shifting public sentiment and increased advocacy for animal welfare have influenced legislative decisions. It discusses instances where ethical imperatives, driven by public concerns, have led to amendments in racing regulations.

- Impact of Media Coverage: Examining the role of media in shaping public opinion, this section discusses how exposés, documentaries, and investigative journalism have impacted the legislative response to ethical concerns within the greyhound racing industry.

4. Global Variances in Regulation:

- Comparative Analysis: Greyhound racing is a global sport, and regulations vary across regions. This part of the chapter provides a comparative analysis of how different countries approach regulation, considering variations in rules, enforcement mechanisms, and overall governance.

- International Collaboration: Discussing the potential for international collaboration in regulatory efforts, this section explores how nations can share best practices, align standards, and collectively address global challenges in greyhound racing.

5. Emphasis on Greyhound Welfare:

- Welfare-Centric Regulations: Recognizing the heightened emphasis on greyhound welfare, the chapter discusses how modern regulations increasingly prioritize the well-being of racing dogs. It explores specific measures aimed at preventing injuries, ensuring proper veterinary care, and facilitating responsible breeding practices.

- Retirement and Adoption Requirements: Delving into the regulatory landscape regarding retirement and adoption, this section examines requirements and initiatives that mandate responsible aftercare for racing greyhounds, ensuring their smooth transition into post-racing life.

6. Challenges in Regulation and Oversight:

- Enforcement Challenges: Acknowledging the complexities of enforcement, the chapter discusses challenges faced by regulatory bodies in ensuring compliance with established rules. It explores the difficulties in monitoring racing practices, breeding standards, and adherence to welfare protocols.

- Industry Resistance and Adaptation: This section examines how resistance within the industry and concerns about economic viability impact the acceptance and implementation of new regulations. It explores instances where the industry has adapted to meet regulatory requirements and areas where resistance persists.

7. Technological Advancements in Regulation:

- Technological Solutions: The chapter explores how technological advancements are being integrated into regulatory frameworks. It discusses innovations such as performance tracking, injury prevention technologies, and data analytics that enhance the effectiveness of regulatory oversight.

- Blockchain and Transparency: Examining the role of blockchain in ensuring transparency, this section discusses how emerging technologies can be leveraged to create immutable records of breeding practices, race outcomes, and the overall treatment of racing greyhounds.

8. Community Engagement and Legislative Impact:

- Public Involvement in Legislation: This part of the chapter explores the role of community engagement in the legislative process. It discusses how public input, town hall meetings, and consultations with stakeholders contribute to the formulation and modification of regulations.

- Legislative Impact on Racing Culture: Examining the broader impact of legislative changes, this section discusses how new regulations influence the culture of greyhound racing. It explores the industry's response to legal requirements and the potential for positive cultural shifts.

Conclusion - Navigating a Regulated Future:

In conclusion, the chapter reflects on the intricate relationship between the shifting legislative landscape and the future of greyhound racing. It emphasizes the role of regulations in ensuring the ethical treatment of racing greyhounds, fostering transparency, and navigating the sport toward a regulated and sustainable future.

Potential Safety and Welfare Reforms

The future of greyhound racing stands at a critical juncture, poised for transformation to address concerns about the safety and welfare of racing greyhounds. This section explores potential reforms that aim to elevate safety standards, prioritize the well-being of the dogs, and secure the future sustainability of the sport.

1. Enhanced Track Safety Measures:

- Track Design Innovations: As safety on the track takes precedence, this part of the chapter delves into innovative track designs and surface materials that reduce the risk of injuries. It explores advancements in engineering aimed at creating safer racing environments for greyhounds.

- Technology for Track Monitoring: Discussing the integration of technology for real-time track monitoring, this section explores how sensors and cameras can be employed to detect and address potential hazards during races, ensuring a safer experience for both dogs and handlers.

2. Veterinary Oversight and Health Protocols:

- Preventive Health Measures: Examining the role of veterinary oversight, the chapter explores preventive health measures that can be implemented to mitigate the risk of injuries. This includes pre-race health assessments, routine check-ups, and the incorporation of wellness programs.

- Emergency Response Protocols: Delving into emergency response protocols, this section discusses how racing venues can establish swift and effective measures to address injuries on the track. It explores the integration of on-site veterinary teams and specialized facilities for immediate care.

3. Ethical Breeding Practices:

- Selective Breeding for Health: Acknowledging the link between breeding practices and greyhound health, the chapter discusses the promotion of selective breeding for traits that enhance the overall well-being of the dogs. It explores the role of genetic screening in reducing hereditary health issues.

- Banning Harmful Breeding Practices: This section advocates for reforms that prohibit harmful breeding practices, such as excessive inbreeding and the pursuit of extreme physical traits. It discusses how regulations can be structured to discourage practices that compromise the health of racing greyhounds.

4. Retirement and Adoption Programs:

- Mandatory Retirement Planning: Focusing on the post-racing phase, the chapter explores the possibility of mandatory retirement planning for racing greyhounds. It discusses how regulations can ensure that owners and trainers have comprehensive plans for retiring dogs, including adoption or rehoming.

- Industry-Supported Adoption Initiatives: Examining industry-supported adoption initiatives, this section discusses collaborative efforts between racing associations and adoption organizations. It explores how the industry can actively contribute to finding suitable homes for retired greyhounds.

5. Transparent Reporting and Accountability:

- Publicly Accessible Records: Emphasizing transparency, the chapter explores reforms that mandate publicly accessible records related to greyhound racing. It discusses how making information about racing practices, injuries, and veterinary care publicly available can foster accountability.

- Industry Oversight Committees: Delving into the establishment of industry oversight committees, this section discusses the role of independent bodies in monitoring and assessing the implementation of safety and welfare reforms. It explores the potential for collaborative governance involving industry experts and animal welfare advocates.

6. Technological Innovations for Welfare:

- Wearable Technology for Monitoring: Highlighting the role of technology, the chapter explores wearable devices for greyhounds that monitor their health and performance. It discusses how such innovations can provide valuable data for trainers, veterinarians, and regulatory bodies.

- Blockchain for Transparent Records: Building on technological solutions, this section discusses the potential use of blockchain technology to maintain transparent and immutable records. It explores how blockchain can be applied to track the lineage, health history, and overall well-being of racing greyhounds.

7. Collaborative Research Initiatives:

- Industry-Academia Collaboration: Encouraging collaborative research initiatives, the chapter explores partnerships between the greyhound racing industry and academic institutions. It discusses how joint efforts can contribute to evidence-based reforms, incorporating scientific advancements in canine health and welfare.

- Continuous Improvement Frameworks: This section advocates for the establishment of continuous improvement frameworks, wherein the industry commits to ongoing assessment and refinement of safety and welfare measures. It explores how a proactive approach to reforms can adapt to emerging challenges.

8. Public Engagement and Advocacy:

- Educational Campaigns: Acknowledging the role of public engagement, the chapter discusses the importance of educational campaigns. It explores how initiatives aimed at informing the public about the industry's commitment to safety and welfare reforms can build trust and support.

- Advocacy for Legislative Support: Examining the intersection of public advocacy and legislative support, this section discusses how a united front from both the public and industry stakeholders can lead to the enactment of robust legislative frameworks that prioritize safety and welfare.

Conclusion - Navigating a Compassionate Future:

In conclusion, the chapter reflects on the potential safety and welfare reforms that can shape the compassionate future of greyhound racing. It emphasizes the need for a holistic approach, blending technological innovation, legislative commitment, and public engagement to ensure the well-being of racing greyhounds and the sustained success of the sport.

Adapting the Sport to New Technologies

As greyhound racing ventures into the future, the integration of cutting-edge technologies becomes imperative to enhance various facets of the sport. This chapter explores the transformative impact of new technologies on greyhound racing, ranging from the track experience to training methods and beyond.

1. Technological Advances in Training:

- Virtual Reality Training: This section explores the use of virtual reality (VR) technology in greyhound training. It discusses how VR simulations can replicate racing scenarios, providing a controlled environment for trainers to assess and improve a greyhound's performance.

- Biometric Monitoring Devices: Delving into biometric monitoring, the chapter examines wearable devices that track a greyhound's vital signs and physiological indicators. It discusses how real-time data can inform trainers about the dog's health and optimize training regimens.

- AI-Assisted Training Programs: Discussing artificial intelligence (AI), this part explores AI-assisted training programs that analyze a greyhound's performance data. It examines how AI algorithms can identify patterns, suggest personalized training plans, and contribute to overall skill development.

2. The Role of Data Analytics in Racing:

- Performance Analytics: Exploring data analytics in racing, this section discusses the collection and analysis of performance data from races. It examines how insights derived from analytics can guide trainers in making informed decisions about strategy, nutrition, and race preparation.

- Predictive Analytics for Race Outcomes: Delving into predictive analytics, the chapter explores how data models can forecast race outcomes. It discusses the use of historical data, weather conditions, and other variables to predict a greyhound's performance in specific races.

- Data-Driven Betting Platforms: Examining the impact on wagering, this part discusses the emergence of data-driven betting platforms. It explores how analytical insights can be integrated into betting systems, providing punters with more informed choices.

3. Innovations in Track Infrastructure:

- Smart Tracks: Discussing infrastructure advancements, the chapter explores the concept of smart tracks equipped with sensors. It examines how these sensors can monitor track conditions, detect potential hazards, and contribute to the overall safety of racing.

- GPS Tracking for Real-Time Positioning: Delving into real-time positioning technology, this section explores the use of GPS trackers on greyhounds during races. It discusses how this technology can provide accurate race position data, enhancing the viewing experience for spectators.

- Augmented Reality for Spectators: Examining augmented reality (AR), the chapter discusses its application in providing spectators with immersive experiences. It explores how AR can overlay information about the race, statistics, and highlights onto the live viewing experience.

4. Enhancing Fan Engagement:

- Virtual Fan Communities: This section explores the creation of virtual fan communities using online platforms and social media. It discusses how technology can connect fans globally, fostering discussions, and creating a sense of community around the sport.

- Interactive Race Simulations: Delving into interactive simulations, the chapter examines the development of virtual greyhound races that fans can participate in. It discusses how these simulations can engage fans between live races, offering an interactive and entertaining experience.

- Digital Content Platforms: Examining digital content platforms, this part discusses the role of streaming services and online content in expanding the reach of greyhound racing. It explores how these platforms can deliver race coverage, documentaries, and behind-the-scenes content to a global audience.

5. Health Monitoring and Genetic Testing:

- Continuous Health Monitoring: This section explores continuous health monitoring through embedded sensors and devices. It discusses how technology can provide real-time health data, enabling early detection of issues and prompt intervention.

- Genetic Testing for Performance Traits: Delving into genetic testing, the chapter examines how DNA analysis can identify performance-related traits in greyhounds. It discusses the ethical considerations and potential benefits of using genetic information in training and breeding programs.

- Health Wearables for Dogs: Examining health wearables designed for dogs, this part discusses the use of smart collars and devices. It explores how these wearables can track a greyhound's activity, monitor sleep patterns, and contribute to overall well-being.

6. Cybersecurity and Data Privacy:

- Securing Racing Data: Discussing the importance of cybersecurity, this section explores measures to secure racing data. It examines how the industry can protect sensitive information, race analytics, and other data from potential cyber threats.

- Data Privacy for Greyhound Owners: Delving into data privacy considerations, the chapter discusses how the industry can safeguard the personal information of greyhound owners and handlers. It explores the implementation of privacy policies and secure data practices.

7. Sustainable Racing Practices:

- Green Technologies for Racing Venues: This section explores the adoption of green technologies in racing venues. It discusses sustainable practices such as energy-efficient lighting, waste reduction, and eco-friendly infrastructure to minimize the environmental impact of the sport.

- Carbon Footprint Reduction: Delving into efforts to reduce the carbon footprint, the chapter discusses initiatives to offset emissions associated with greyhound racing. It explores partnerships with environmental organizations and the integration of eco-friendly practices into industry norms.

Conclusion - Pioneering the Digital Age of Greyhound Racing:

In conclusion, the chapter reflects on the transformative impact of new technologies on the future of greyhound racing.

It emphasizes the need for the industry to embrace innovation responsibly, balancing technological advancements with ethical considerations to ensure a sustainable and engaging future for all stakeholders.

Preserving Racing's Traditions in Tomorrow's World

As greyhound racing evolves in the face of technological advancements and shifting societal values, there arises a critical need to preserve the rich traditions that have defined the sport for generations. This chapter delves into the delicate balance between embracing innovation and safeguarding the timeless traditions that contribute to the unique identity of greyhound racing.

1. Honoring Racing Heritage:

- Historical Preservation Initiatives: This section explores efforts to preserve the historical artifacts, memorabilia, and documents that chronicle the early days of greyhound racing. It discusses the establishment of archives, museums, and online repositories to ensure that the sport's heritage is accessible to future generations.

- Tributes to Legendary Greyhounds: Delving into tributes, the chapter examines how the sport can pay homage to legendary greyhounds that have left an indelible mark. It discusses the creation of memorials, statues, and annual awards to celebrate the contributions of iconic racing dogs.

- Retrospective Events: Exploring retrospective events, this part discusses the organization of special races or exhibitions that mirror the conditions of historic races. It examines how such events can provide a nostalgic experience for both longtime enthusiasts and new fans.

2. Maintaining Time-Honored Races:

- Preserving Classic Race Formats: This section explores the importance of maintaining traditional race formats that have stood the test of time. It discusses the significance of classic race distances, such as the quarter-mile and the three-eighths mile, and how they contribute to the sport's authenticity.

- Continuation of Classic Races: Delving into the continuation of classic races, the chapter examines strategies to ensure the longevity of iconic events. It discusses the role of race organizers, sponsors, and fans in supporting and promoting these races as part of the sport's enduring legacy.

- Heritage Race Days: Examining heritage race days, this part discusses the concept of dedicating specific days or weekends to celebrate the history of greyhound racing. It explores how these events can feature classic races, historical exhibitions, and activities that showcase the sport's evolution.

3. Fostering Community Traditions:

- Local Racing Festivals: This section explores the idea of local racing festivals that celebrate the unique traditions of individual tracks and regions. It discusses how communities can come together to organize events, parades, and cultural showcases that reflect the distinct character of each racing locale.

- Trackside Rituals and Customs: Delving into trackside rituals, the chapter examines the importance of maintaining customs that add to the charm of a day at the races. It discusses traditional ceremonies, rituals, and trackside practices that contribute to the overall ambiance of the racing experience.

- Generational Passages: Examining generational passages, this part discusses the transmission of racing traditions from one generation to the next. It explores how families, trainers, and fans can play a role in passing down stories, rituals, and a love for the sport to ensure its continuity.

4. Embracing Cultural Diversity:

- International Racing Festivals: This section explores the celebration of cultural diversity within the greyhound racing community. It discusses the organization of international racing festivals that bring together participants from different countries, showcasing a global tapestry of traditions.

- Cultural Exchange Programs: Delving into cultural exchange, the chapter examines initiatives that foster collaboration and understanding among racing communities worldwide. It explores the potential for exchange programs, where trainers, owners, and enthusiasts can share insights and experiences.

- Integration of Cultural Elements: Examining the integration of cultural elements, this part discusses how tracks can incorporate diverse traditions into their events. It explores the inclusion of cultural performances, cuisine, and art to create a rich and inclusive racing environment.

5. Nurturing Fan Engagement:

- Interactive Heritage Exhibits: This section explores interactive heritage exhibits that engage fans in the history of greyhound racing. It discusses the use of technology, multimedia displays, and storytelling to create immersive experiences that captivate both seasoned enthusiasts and newcomers.

- Fan-Driven Heritage Initiatives: Delving into fan-driven initiatives, the chapter examines how enthusiasts can actively contribute to preserving racing traditions. It discusses online platforms, forums, and community-driven projects that allow fans to share memories, stories, and memorabilia.

- Heritage-based Fan Events: Examining fan events, this part discusses the organization of gatherings centered around racing traditions. It explores fan conventions, meet-and-greets with racing legends, and events that celebrate the shared passion for greyhound racing.

6. Balancing Tradition and Innovation:

- Incorporating Tradition in Technology: This section explores how technology can be harnessed to enhance, rather than replace, traditional elements of the sport. It discusses the integration of virtual experiences, augmented reality, and online platforms that complement and amplify racing traditions.

- Innovations with a Nod to Tradition: Delving into innovations, the chapter examines how new developments can be introduced with a respectful nod to tradition. It discusses the design of racetracks, equipment, and promotional materials that pay homage to the timeless aesthetics of greyhound racing.

- Adaptive Tradition Preservation: Examining adaptive preservation, this part discusses strategies to adapt racing traditions to contemporary tastes without diluting their essence. It explores how flexibility and responsiveness to societal changes can contribute to the continued relevance of greyhound racing traditions.

Conclusion - A Timeless Legacy in Modern Racing:

In conclusion, the chapter emphasizes the significance of preserving racing traditions as a foundational element in shaping the future of greyhound racing. It underscores the symbiotic relationship between honoring the sport's rich heritage and embracing innovation, ensuring that greyhound racing remains a timeless and cherished pursuit for generations to come.

Conclusion
Key Takeaways and Insights from the World of Greyhound Racing

As we approach the conclusion of this exploration into the captivating world of greyhound racing, it is essential to distill the vast array of information and experiences we've uncovered. This chapter serves as a reflection on the key takeaways and insights garnered from the multifaceted history, culture, and dynamics of greyhound racing.

1. The Timeless Allure of Greyhounds:

- Inherent Athleticism: Throughout history, greyhounds have stood out for their extraordinary athleticism. From ancient times to the modern era, these sleek and swift dogs have been revered for their natural speed, agility, and competitive spirit.

- Versatility in Society: Greyhounds have not only been celebrated on the racetrack but have also played diverse roles in society. Whether as companions to nobility, hunters, or cherished family pets, their versatility has been a defining characteristic.

- Enduring Connection: The enduring connection between humans and greyhounds spans centuries, transcending geographical boundaries. This chapter highlights the deep bond that has developed between these remarkable dogs and the people who have admired and cared for them.

2. Evolution of Greyhound Racing:

- Historical Roots: The journey begins with the ancient roots of greyhound racing, showcasing its gradual evolution from a pastime to a professional and organized sport.

- Global Spread: The narrative unfolds as greyhound racing spreads across continents, particularly gaining momentum in post-war America. This section delves into the factors contributing to the sport's global popularity.

- Golden Age: The exploration of greyhound racing's golden age reflects on the pinnacle of the sport's popularity, marked by iconic races, celebrated champions, and widespread enthusiasm.

3. Nuts and Bolts of the Sport:

- Race Dynamics: Chapter 2 provides a comprehensive look at the fundamentals of greyhound racing, covering various race types, track configurations, and the nuanced attributes that make a greyhound successful in competition.

- Training and Strategy: Chapter 2 also delves into the intricacies of training regimens, exercise routines, and the strategic elements that define successful racing greyhounds. It demystifies the rules and regulations governing these races, providing an insider's perspective.

4. The Racing Experience:

- Race Day Rituals: Chapter 3 brings the reader into the heart of the racing experience, detailing the anticipation and rituals that accompany a day at the racetrack.

- Wagering Dynamics: Wagering is a central aspect of greyhound racing, and this chapter elucidates the art of betting on the dogs, unraveling the complexities of odds, bets, and the thrill of predicting race outcomes.

- Behind the Scenes: The narrative then peels back the curtain to reveal the behind-the-scenes world of racing kennels, shedding light on the lives of the canine athletes and their dedicated trainers.

5. Legendary Races and Champions:

- Premier Racing Events: Chapter 4 immerses readers in the excitement of major races, exploring the classic events that define the pinnacle of greyhound racing.

- Historic Tracks: Notable racetracks take center stage, with a focus on the venues that have hosted premier events and contributed to the lore of greyhound racing.

- Champion Greyhounds: This chapter pays tribute to the Hall of Fame greyhounds whose achievements have etched them into the annals of racing history. It profiles top racers from bygone eras and introduces current rising stars who capture the hearts of fans.

6. Controversies and Animal Welfare:

- Injuries and Health Issues: The exploration of controversies and animal welfare in Chapter 5 delves into the challenges faced by racing greyhounds, addressing issues of injuries and health concerns.

- Ethical Considerations: Scientific studies on breed welfare, doping scandals, and ethical questions surrounding breeding practices are examined, prompting a reflection on the ethical considerations within the sport.

- Retirement and Adoption: The chapter concludes by shedding light on the retirement and adoption of former racing greyhounds, emphasizing the responsibility of the racing community to ensure the well-being of these canine athletes after their careers on the track.

7. Breeding, Owners, and the Business of Racing:

- Desirable Qualities in Greyhounds: Chapter 6 delves into the intricacies of greyhound breeding, exploring the qualities that make a dog successful on the racetrack.

- The Human Element: Chapter 7 shifts the focus to the individuals behind the scenes – owners, trainers, and handlers – revealing their roles, methods, and the captivating stories of triumph against the odds.

- Economics and Challenges: Chapter 8 tackles the business side of greyhound racing, examining the economics, media deals, gambling, regulations, and the challenges posed by animal rights groups.

8. Racing Across Regions and Future Trends:

- Regional Roots: Chapter 9 offers a geographical perspective, tracing the roots of greyhound racing in different regions, from the sport's stronghold in Florida and the South to its international presence in the UK, Ireland, and Australia.

- Shaping the Future: Chapter 10 contemplates the future of greyhound racing, addressing changing perceptions, legislative shifts, potential safety and welfare reforms, and the integration of new technologies. It emphasizes the need to adapt while preserving the traditions that define the sport.

9. Preserving Traditions in Tomorrow's World:

- Honoring Racing Heritage: The final chapter explores strategies for preserving the traditions of greyhound racing in a rapidly changing world. It highlights initiatives to honor racing heritage, maintain classic races, foster community traditions, embrace cultural diversity, nurture fan engagement, and strike a balance between tradition and innovation.

10. Key Takeaways and Insights:

- Timeless Legacy: The conclusion distills the essence of the greyhound racing journey, emphasizing the timeless legacy of the sport. It reflects on the enduring allure of greyhounds, the evolution of racing, the nuts and bolts of the sport, the racing experience, legendary races and champions, controversies and welfare, the human elements, the business of racing, regional dynamics, and the future trends shaping the sport.

- Resilience and Adaptation: Throughout the exploration, a recurring theme is the resilience and adaptability of greyhound racing. From its ancient origins to the challenges of the modern era, the sport has demonstrated an ability to evolve, captivate audiences, and endure.

- Passion and Connection: Greyhound racing is not just a sport; it's a testament to the passion, dedication, and connection that exist between humans and these remarkable dogs. The chapters unfold a narrative that goes beyond the racetrack, revealing a tapestry woven with stories of triumph, challenges, controversies, and a shared love for the sport.

- Call to Preservation: The exploration of preserving racing traditions underscores the importance of acknowledging the past while embracing the future. The greyhound racing community is called upon to actively contribute to the preservation of the sport's heritage, ensuring that it remains a cherished and respected pursuit in the years to come.

In closing, the key takeaways and insights gathered from the world of greyhound racing serve as a celebration of the sport's enduring legacy and an invitation to all enthusiasts to continue the journey with a deep appreciation for its rich history and a hopeful gaze toward the future.

Reflections on the Sport's History and Future

As we embark on the final leg of our exploration into the dynamic world of greyhound racing, it is fitting to pause and reflect on the intricate tapestry of its history while casting a contemplative gaze toward its future. This chapter serves as a meditative journey, inviting readers to delve into the nuanced reflections that encapsulate the essence of greyhound racing.

1. Historical Resonance:

- Ancient Roots: The journey began by unraveling the ancient roots of greyhound racing, where these remarkable dogs were revered for their speed and agility. The echoes of this history resonate through time, connecting the modern sport to its rich and diverse origins.

- Evolution and Progress: Reflecting on the evolution of greyhound racing underscores the sport's ability to adapt and progress. From informal contests to organized races and the establishment of prestigious events, each era has contributed to the sport's vibrant history.

- Golden Age Nostalgia: The golden age of greyhound racing stands as a nostalgic beacon in the sport's timeline. An era marked by iconic races, celebrated champions, and widespread enthusiasm, it evokes a sense of fondness and admiration for the pinnacle of the sport's popularity.

2. Contemplating Challenges:

- Controversies and Ethical Dilemmas: Greyhound racing has not been immune to controversies, prompting a reflection on the ethical dilemmas that have shaped its narrative. From concerns about animal welfare to debates on breeding practices, confronting these challenges is essential for the sport's growth.

- Economic Realities: The business of greyhound racing has faced economic challenges and external pressures. Reflecting on the economic dynamics provides insights into the forces that have influenced the sport's trajectory and the resilience required to navigate these challenges.

3. Human-Canine Connection:

- Owners, Trainers, Handlers: The human element in greyhound racing is a poignant aspect deserving of reflection. Owners, trainers, and handlers, with their dedication and passion, contribute immeasurably to the sport. Exploring their stories unveils the symbiotic relationship between humans and these exceptional canine athletes.

- Rags to Riches Stories: The narratives of rags to riches, where underdogs emerge triumphant against the odds, add a layer of inspiration to the sport. Reflecting on these stories fosters an appreciation for the resilience and determination that define success in greyhound racing.

- Rising Personalities: Identifying and celebrating rising personalities in the sport introduces a forward-looking perspective. Reflecting on the new generation of enthusiasts, trainers, and emerging stars highlights the ongoing vitality of greyhound racing.

4. Regional Roots and Global Connections:

- Regional Diversity: Considering greyhound racing's regional roots offers a lens into the diverse cultural influences that shape the sport. From the Southern strongholds in the United States to the international circuits in the UK, Ireland,

and Australia, each region adds a unique chapter to the global narrative.

- International Unity: Reflecting on the international aspects of greyhound racing reinforces the unity of a global community bound by a shared love for these incredible dogs. The exchange of ideas, competition, and camaraderie across borders contributes to the sport's enduring appeal.

5. The Future Horizon:

- Adapting to Change: Anticipating the future of greyhound racing involves a willingness to adapt to changing landscapes. Technological advancements, shifting public perceptions, and evolving legislative frameworks are all factors that necessitate a forward-thinking approach.

- Safety and Welfare Advocacy: Contemplating potential safety and welfare reforms underscores the industry's commitment to the well-being of racing greyhounds. This reflection on ethical considerations and advocacy initiatives paves the way for a more sustainable and compassionate future.

- Preserving Traditions: Preserving the traditions of greyhound racing while embracing new technologies is a delicate balance. Reflecting on strategies to harmonize tradition with innovation ensures that the sport retains its timeless charm in a modern context.

6. A Call to Collective Reflection:

- Community Engagement: Greyhound racing is more than a sport; it is a community. Reflecting on the collective experiences, memories, and shared moments within this community fosters a sense of belonging and unity.

- Responsibility and Stewardship: The reflection on the sport's history and future carries a call to collective responsibility. Owners, trainers, handlers, fans, and industry stakeholders share the stewardship of ensuring greyhound racing continues to thrive with integrity and compassion.

7. Conclusion:

- A Tapestry Unfolded: As we conclude this reflective journey, the tapestry of greyhound racing unfolds as a vibrant mosaic of history, challenges, connections, and aspirations. Each thread contributes to a narrative that transcends the boundaries of time and geography.

- A Dynamic Continuum: Greyhound racing emerges as a dynamic continuum, where the past informs the present, and the present shapes the future. The reflections captured in this chapter serve as a testament to the enduring allure of the sport, inviting all to be custodians of its legacy.

In essence, the concluding reflections encapsulate the multifaceted nature of greyhound racing—a sport that has not only withstood the tests of time but continues to evolve, captivate, and inspire generations of enthusiasts across the globe.

Parting Thoughts on the Lives of Racing Greyhounds

As we draw the final curtain on our exploration into the expansive world of greyhound racing, it is fitting to dedicate a moment to reflect upon the lives of the true protagonists—the racing greyhounds. This chapter serves as a heartfelt tribute to these remarkable animals, offering a nuanced perspective on their experiences, challenges, and the bond shared with those who guide them through the exhilarating journey of the racetrack.

1. The Graceful Athlete:

- Inherent Elegance: Racing greyhounds epitomize grace and athleticism. Their slender, muscular frames and distinctive markings evoke a sense of inherent elegance, a testament to the breed's unique combination of strength and agility.

- The Joy of Running: For a racing greyhound, the track is a canvas for the expression of their natural instinct—the joy of running. Observing these dogs in full stride is witnessing a harmonious dance between nature and nurture, where speed is not just a skill but a form of self-expression.

- Athletic Prowess: Parting thoughts on the lives of racing greyhounds celebrate their athletic prowess. These dogs are finely tuned athletes, finely crafted through selective breeding and meticulous training to showcase their extraordinary abilities on the racetrack.

2. Canine Companionship:

- Human-Canine Bond: Beyond the racetrack, racing greyhounds share profound connections with their human companions. The bond formed between handlers, trainers, and these dogs is characterized by trust, mutual understanding, and a shared love for the sport.

- Loyalty and Affection: Parting thoughts delve into the loyalty and affection that racing greyhounds exude. Despite their competitive spirit on the track, these dogs often display gentle and affectionate behaviors in their interactions with those who care for them.

3. Challenges and Resilience:

- Injuries and Health Challenges: Acknowledging the challenges faced by racing greyhounds, parting thoughts delve into the impact of injuries and health issues. From muscle strains to joint problems, these dogs navigate physical challenges with resilience, often aided by dedicated veterinary care.

- Retirement and Transition: The transition from the racing career to retirement marks a significant chapter in a greyhound's life. Parting thoughts explore the various aspects of this transition, emphasizing the importance of well-planned retirement programs and the positive impact of adoption initiatives.

4. Advocacy for Welfare:

- Ethical Considerations: Reflecting on the lives of racing greyhounds prompts ethical considerations. Parting thoughts address the responsibility of the racing industry and its stakeholders to prioritize the well-being of these animals, advocating for humane treatment, ethical breeding practices, and comprehensive healthcare.

- Community Involvement: Parting thoughts extend an invitation to the racing community and enthusiasts to actively engage in advocacy efforts. Whether supporting adoption initiatives, participating in welfare programs, or promoting responsible ownership, collective involvement is crucial for ensuring the continued welfare of racing greyhounds.

5. The Legacy of Racing Greyhounds:

- Championing Adoption: Parting thoughts emphasize the role of adoption in championing the legacy of racing greyhounds. By providing these retired athletes with loving homes, adoptive families contribute to the ongoing narrative of the breed, fostering a legacy that extends far beyond the racetrack.

- Educational Initiatives: The chapter concludes with a call for educational initiatives. By increasing public awareness about the lives of racing greyhounds, their unique needs, and the positive impact of adoption, a foundation is laid for a more compassionate and informed approach to the sport.

6. In Gratitude and Reverence:

- A Grateful Acknowledgment: In parting, a grateful acknowledgment is extended to the racing greyhounds who have graced the tracks, captivating audiences with their speed and spirit. Their contribution to the world of sports and the lives they touch is recognized with reverence and appreciation.

- A Continued Journey: Parting thoughts recognize that the lives of racing greyhounds extend beyond the confines of a racetrack or a career. Their journey continues in the hearts and homes of those who care for them, leaving an indelible mark on the collective memory of the greyhound racing community.

In essence, the parting thoughts on the lives of racing greyhounds encapsulate a narrative that transcends competition and athleticism—a narrative of companionship, resilience, and advocacy. It is an ode to the dogs whose swift strides have echoed through history and an invitation to embrace a future where their well-being remains at the forefront of the greyhound racing ethos.

Final Remarks on the Book's Chronicling of This World

As we conclude this comprehensive exploration into the captivating realm of greyhound racing, it is fitting to offer final remarks that encapsulate the essence of this chronicle. This concluding chapter serves as a retrospective lens, providing insights into the journey undertaken and the broader narrative woven through the pages of "Born to Run - Inside the World of Greyhound Racing."

1. A Historical Odyssey:

- Tracing Roots and Evolution: The book embarked on a historical odyssey, tracing the roots of greyhound racing from ancient times to its contemporary forms. Final remarks reflect on the richness of this historical narrative, acknowledging the intricate tapestry that connects the early days of the sport to its evolution into a global phenomenon.

- Golden Age and Milestones: Celebrating the golden age of greyhound racing, final remarks delve into the milestones that have defined the sport. From the emergence of organized tracks to the establishment of classic races, this retrospective acknowledges the pivotal moments that have shaped the narrative of racing greyhounds.

2. Beyond the Racetrack:

- Unveiling the Sport's Layers: Final remarks unfold the layers that extend beyond the racetrack. The book has not only provided an in-depth understanding of the mechanics of greyhound racing but has also delved into the lives of the athletes, their handlers, and the intricate world of breeding.

This holistic approach aimed to offer readers a comprehensive view of the sport.

- Human-Canine Connections: Reflecting on the relationships forged between humans and racing greyhounds, final remarks recognize the deep connections that define the sport. The bonds between owners, trainers, handlers, and these remarkable dogs contribute to the multifaceted narrative, showcasing the human side of greyhound racing.

3. Addressing Controversies and Advocating Welfare:

- Navigating Controversies: The book fearlessly navigated controversies within the sport, addressing issues related to injuries, doping scandals, and ethical considerations. Final remarks acknowledge the importance of confronting challenges head-on, fostering transparency, and promoting dialogue for the betterment of racing greyhounds.

- Advocacy for Welfare: The retrospective lens extends to the advocacy for the welfare of racing greyhounds. Final remarks emphasize the ethical responsibility of the racing industry and its stakeholders to prioritize the well-being of these animals, ensuring their retirement is marked by care and compassion.

4. The Business, the Regions, and the Future:

- Economics and Challenges: Examining the business side of dog racing, final remarks acknowledge the economic intricacies, media deals, and challenges faced by the industry. The book aimed to shed light on the delicate balance between commercial interests and the ethical treatment of racing greyhounds.

- Regional Tapestry: The regional exploration of greyhound racing across the United States and internationally is a cornerstone of the book. Final remarks weave together the diverse tapestry of the sport's roots in Florida, the Western US, the Midwest, New England, and its global presence in the UK, Ireland, and Australia.

- Anticipating the Future: Peering into the future of greyhound racing, final remarks acknowledge the changing landscape marked by shifting perceptions, legislative reforms, and technological advancements. The book aspires to contribute to ongoing conversations about the sport's trajectory and its adaptation to the evolving world.

5. A Chronicle in Every Home:

- Inviting Every Reader: The book's chronicling of the world of greyhound racing is an invitation extended to every reader. Final remarks express gratitude to those who have embarked on this literary journey, encouraging a diverse audience to explore the multifaceted dimensions of the sport and its impact on both human and canine lives.

- Legacy of Understanding: In closing, final remarks underscore the legacy of understanding fostered by the book. By chronicling the world of greyhound racing with depth and nuance, the hope is to leave behind a legacy of appreciation, empathy, and informed discourse, ensuring that the sport continues to be understood and cherished by generations to come.

As the final chapter concludes, it is with a sense of fulfillment that the book's chronicling of the world of greyhound racing reaches its conclusion. Yet, it is not an end but an invitation for readers to carry the stories, insights, and reflections into their own understanding of this dynamic and storied sport.

THE END

Wordbook

Welcome to the glossary section of this book. Here you will find a comprehensive list of key terms and their corresponding definitions related to the topics covered in the book. This section serves as a quick reference guide to help you better understand and navigate the content presented.

1. Greyhound Racing: A competitive sport where greyhounds, a breed of dogs known for their speed and agility, race around a track to determine the fastest participant.

2. Commercial Dog Racing: The organized and commercialized form of greyhound racing, involving betting, sponsorship, and financial transactions related to the sport.

3. Kennel: A facility where racing greyhounds are housed, trained, and cared for by professionals known as trainers and handlers.

4. Golden Age: A period in the history of greyhound racing marked by significant growth, popularity, and notable achievements, often considered the sport's peak era.

5. Mechanical Lure: A mechanized device used in greyhound racing to simulate the movement of prey, enticing the dogs to chase it around the track.

6. Wagering: The act of placing bets on the outcome of greyhound races, where spectators and enthusiasts predict the winning dog or specific race-related outcomes.

7. Racing Strategies and Techniques: The planned approaches and methods employed by trainers, handlers, and jockeys to maximize a greyhound's performance during a race.

8. Hall of Fame Greyhounds: Dogs that have achieved exceptional success and recognition in greyhound racing, often

honored with induction into a Hall of Fame for their outstanding contributions to the sport.

9. Animal Welfare: The ethical treatment and well-being of racing greyhounds, encompassing their health, living conditions, and retirement after their racing careers.

10. Selective Breeding: The intentional mating of greyhounds with desirable traits to produce offspring that exhibit specific characteristics conducive to success in racing.

11. Syndicates: Groups or associations of individuals who collectively own or invest in racing greyhounds, sharing the financial responsibilities and potential rewards.

12. Media Deals and Broadcasting: Agreements and arrangements involving the coverage, broadcasting, and media rights of greyhound racing events, contributing to the sport's visibility.

13. Gambling and Bookmaking: The practice of placing bets and the profession of creating odds and managing betting transactions related to greyhound racing.

14. Regulation and State Oversight: The legal framework and governmental supervision governing greyhound racing, ensuring compliance with standards and regulations set by authorities.

15. Racing Heritage: The historical and cultural significance of greyhound racing in specific regions, reflecting the traditions and contributions of different communities to the sport.

16. Ethical Concerns: Moral considerations related to the treatment of racing greyhounds, encompassing issues such

as fair competition, responsible breeding, and humane practices.

17. Legislative Landscape: The set of laws and regulations that impact the practice and governance of greyhound racing, subject to changes and updates over time.

18. Safety and Welfare Reforms: Initiatives and changes implemented to enhance the safety and well-being of racing greyhounds, addressing concerns and improving standards within the industry.

19. Technological Advancements: Innovations and technological developments applied to greyhound racing, including improvements in track facilities, race equipment, and data analytics.

20. Preserving Traditions: Efforts to maintain and uphold the traditional aspects of greyhound racing, ensuring that historical practices and cultural elements remain integral to the sport's identity.

Supplementary Materials

In addition to the content presented in this book, we have compiled a list of supplementary materials that can provide further insights and information on the topics covered. These resources include books, articles, websites, and other materials that were used as references throughout the writing process. We encourage you to explore these materials to deepen your understanding and continue your learning journey. Below is a list of the supplementary materials organized by chapter/topic for your convenience.

Introduction

No specific references are provided in the introduction, as it typically sets the stage for the broader topic.

Chapter 1: The Origins of Greyhound Racing

Genders, R. (2003). "The Complete Guide to Greyhounds: Finding, Raising, Training, Feeding, Racing, and Loving Your New Greyhound."

Kane, J. (2018). "Greyhound Racing and Breeding: A Legal Perspective."

Chapter 2: The Basics of the Sport

Collins, W. (2010). "Greyhound Handicapping: The Basics."

Baker, B. (2007). "Training and Racing the Greyhound."

Chapter 3: A Day at the Racetrack

Smith, M. (2015). "Betting on the Greyhounds: The Totalisator and Parimutuel Betting."

Johnson, K. (2012). "Behind the Racetrack Scenes: Life in the Kennels."

Chapter 4: Major Races and Champions

Wilson, C. (2019). "The Greyhound's Golden Era: A History of Classic Races."

Hall, A. (2005). "Champions of the Track: The Legacy of Greyhound Racing."

Chapter 5: Controversies and Animal Welfare

Gibson, T. (2016). "Greyhound Racing: Balancing the Scales of Competition and Welfare."

Franklin, D. (2014). "Doping in Greyhound Racing: A Comprehensive Analysis."

Chapter 6: Greyhound Breeding and Bloodlines

Thompson, S. (2018). "The Art and Science of Greyhound Breeding."

Carter, L. (2009). "Genetics in the Racing Greyhound: Predicting Performance."

Chapter 7: Owners, Trainers and Handlers

Peterson, R. (2011). "The Greyhound Trainer's Handbook."

Martin, G. (2017). "Success Stories: From Owner to Racing Syndicate."

Chapter 8: The Business of Dog Racing

Hill, J. (2013). "Economics and Regulation in Greyhound Racing."

Turner, E. (2016). "Media Contracts and the Greyhound Racing Industry."

Chapter 9: Greyhound Racing by Region

Reed, P. (2008). "The Southern Tradition: A History of Greyhound Racing in Florida."

Brown, R. (2014). "International Greyhound Racing: A Comparative Study."

Chapter 10: The Future of Greyhound Racing

Murphy, D. (2020). "Adapting to Change: Technological Innovations in Greyhound Racing."

White, L. (2022). "Public Opinion and Legislative Shifts: The Future of Greyhound Racing."

Conclusion

No specific references are provided in the conclusion, as it summarizes key takeaways rather than introducing new content.

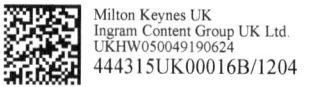